JENNY RUHL

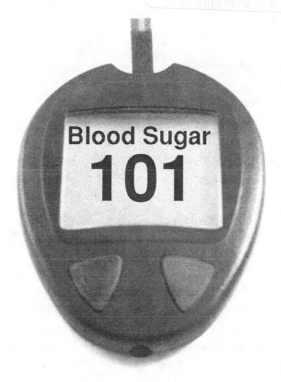

Blood Sugar
101

What They Don't Tell You About **Diabetes**

TECHNION Books

Published by Technion Books
P.O. Box 402
Turners Falls, MA 01376
technion@phlaunt.com

This publication is sold with the understanding that the publisher and author are not engaged in rendering medical or other professional services. **If medical advice or other expert assistance is required, the services of a competent professional person should be sought.**

ISBN-13: 978-0-9647116-1-7
ISBN-10: 0-9647116-1-3

Printed in the United States of America
10 9 8 7 6 5 4 3 2 1

Table of Contents

Introduction

Type 2 Diabetes is a terrible disease. It causes impotence, blindness, kidney failure, amputation, and heart attack death.

But Type 2 Diabetes is also a wonderful disease because all these dreadful outcomes are optional. No matter how severe your diabetes might be at diagnosis, it is unique among the serious chronic diseases in that it is the *only* condition where you, the patient, with only a small amount of help from your doctor and no heroic medical interventions can achieve normal health.

This is probably not what you have heard from your doctors. They probably told you it is *normal* for someone with diabetes to suffer foot pain, impotence, slow wound healing, low physical energy, and even a heart attack. So why should you believe me when I tell you it isn't true?

For a very good reason: Over the past decade diabetes treatment has been revolutionized by the emergence of what is often called "The Wisdom of the Web." This term refers to the phenomenon where many thousands of people, each drawing on their own knowledge and experience, create information resources as good or better than those produced by so-called authorities.

Diabetes on the Web

Diabetes was one of the first diseases to benefit from the Wisdom of the Web because people with diabetes have always been expected to do most of the work involved in managing their disease. They've tested their own blood sugar. They've adjusted their own insulin doses. So even before the advent of the Web they had a lot of information about how their blood sugar responded to changes in their diet, medications, and exercise. What they didn't have was any idea of how their own experience might compare with that of others.

With the emergence of the Web, people with diabetes began to talk to each other on newsgroups and discussion forums, they exchanged information they'd gotten from their solitary testing, they started comparing notes. When they did this, they soon discovered that they weren't the only ones who were having problems with the diets and drug regimens prescribed by doctors and dietitians.

Some people who were active on the Web started trying out alternative diets and drug regimens and reporting their results to each other in the discussion groups. Others started combing through the thousands of peer-reviewed journal articles that had been made available for free on the Web, searching for studies that might point to more effective diabetes treatments. Over time, the information they found and shared started making big improvements in their health.

The 5% Club

Since my own diabetes diagnosis in 1998 I have participated in thousands of Web discussions with hundreds of people with diabetes. Many of them had science or engineering backgrounds like my own.* This gave them a penchant for critical thinking and the skills needed to read and understand journal research. Working together, we learned that it *is* possible for people with diabetes to achieve normal blood sugars. We also uncovered research that suggests that if we maintain truly normal blood sugars we will avoid or even reverse the terrible complications our doctors told us were inevitable.

Some of us call ourselves "The 5% Club" because our goal is to keep our A1c test results under 6%. That is the level most doctors consider to be the normal range. Using a selection of techniques I've learned from participating in Web discussion groups, I've managed to stay in The 5% Club for almost all of the ten years that have followed my diagnosis. Though it has been that long since I was diagnosed, my endocrinologist still refers to me as "recently diagnosed" because she is used to seeing A1cs that low only in people who are new to diabetes.

Why This Book?

Five years ago, after realizing that many people were unaware of the wealth of information to be found in Web discussion groups, I decided to put the most important information on a Web site where people doing Google searches could easily find it. The heart of my Web site was what I learned after spending several months reading through medical

---

* I'm a software developer.

journals, hunting for studies that answered two questions: "What is a truly normal blood sugar level?" and "What blood sugar levels cause organ damage?" The result was my Web site **Bloodsugar101.com**.

This site is different from most other diabetes Web sites because the information you find on it includes links to studies published in top-rated peer-reviewed medical journals. Visitors to the site don't have to take anything on trust. They can follow the links and read the research papers themselves. My Web site is also updated any time something significant turns up in the medical news that is relevant to a topic discussed on its pages.

Over the five years of its existence, the site has grown huge. Visitors started asking me if I could put the mass of information stored on the Web site into book form so they could read it more easily. They explained that because the site has grown so large, they could not read the whole thing on the Web and worried that they might be missing out on critical pieces of information buried in its pages.

Since I had already published seven previous books of nonfiction, including a business bestseller, I was excited by the challenge of turning the site into a book. My enthusiasm for the project grew when I began to write it, as I began to see another advantage to putting what I'd written about diabetes into book form: A book is better than a Web site at explaining ideas that can't be compressed into a few simple paragraphs, because the sequential structure of a book ensures that every concept you encounter in its pages builds on what you have already read. A book is also free of the distractions inherent in the Web's hypertextual design.

So I hope that this book will add value to the Web site by providing, in a compact and portable form, an orderly examination of the crucial concepts that pervade it. In its pages you will find the explanations that will make you understand, as you never have before, how your blood sugar works, what happens when your blood sugar control breaks down, what blood sugar levels damage your organs, and how you can safely lower your blood sugar enough to prevent any further diabetic complications from occurring.

Every concept presented in the text is backed up by peer-reviewed research papers that were published in highly regarded medical journals. If you want check out this research, you can find the citations in the "References" section at the end of this book. You can find links to these studies and the lastest new findings on **Bloodsugar101.com**.

There are some very important issues that people with diabetes must deal with that are not discussed in peer-reviewed research. Here the Wisdom of the Web comes into play, and I draw on the experiences reported by the hundreds of knowledgeable people with diabetes who post messages on the Web. When I cite this type of information, I make it clear that anecdotal reports are its source.

No One Way

Unlike most other diabetes books on the market, this book does not tell you what to eat or what medications to take. If there is one thing we have learned from the Wisdom of the Web, it is that each of us is different and that a strategy that works well for one person may not work for another.

Instead we will teach you how to tell if *any* diabetes strategy you are using is working. By "working" we mean giving you blood sugars low enough to prevent any further organ damage. We'll show you how to find out if your current diabetes diet is doing the job and, if it isn't, we'll show you how to improve it. If you need more than a change of diet to get your blood sugars back into the safe zone, we'll explore what the diabetes drugs available to you are good for and what their drawbacks are, putting particular emphasis on some cheap but effective diabetes drugs that doctors may overlook because they aren't being promoted by drug company marketing campaigns.

What's in it for You?

When you are done reading this book, you will know enough to hold an intelligent conversation with your doctor about your treatment choices. You'll be better able to evaluate the latest "breakthroughs" you read about in the diabetes news. And most importantly, you'll have the information you need to keep yourself safe, no matter what current fad is sweeping the medical community. In short, when you are done with this book, you will have the tools you will need to join "The 5% Club" yourself. So welcome aboard!

Chapter One
What is Normal Blood Sugar?

Diabetes is not a disease, it is a symptom.

Everyone diagnosed with any type of diabetes shares a single symptom with every other person with diabetes. That symptom is high blood sugar.

Anything that interferes with the complex mechanisms that the body uses to regulate blood sugar may cause diabetes. It may occur when the cells that secrete insulin get poisoned or die off or when those cells fail to respond to the signals that tell them to make insulin. It may even occur when those cells are making plenty of insulin but insulin receptors in the cells have lost their ability to respond to it. Diabetes can be caused by abnormalities of the adrenal glands or problems with hormones in the gut that inform the body of the presence of food.

It is also possible for one person to have more than one of these metabolic problems at the same time. For example, the most common form of diabetes, which doctors call Type 2 Diabetes, is frequently described as being caused by insulin resistance, the condition where cell receptors stop responding properly to insulin. But scientists have recently discovered that almost one in twelve of those diagnosed with insulin resistant Type 2 Diabetes also have markers in their bloodstream that show they have been the victim of an autoimmune attack that has killed off the cells that make insulin.

What does this mean for you?

Simply this: Though you may have been diagnosed with diabetes, all that your diabetes, my diabetes, and the diabetes of the person sitting across from you at the diabetes support group meeting have in common is that they cause all of us to have abnormally high blood sugars. The cause of our high blood sugars may be different, how high our blood sugars rise after we eat the identical meal may be different, how our bodies respond to the same dose of the same drug may be dramatically different, and, most importantly, what it takes to bring our blood sugars back into the normal range that prevents complications will be different.

Because we are all so different, the key to recovering good health is to figure out how your own individual version of diabetes works. The first step towards doing this is to learn how blood sugar is regulated in a normal person and how normal blood sugar control breaks down. Armed with this information you will be better able to understand what the various interventions used to treat diabetes do—and which ones might be right for you. So take the time to understand the information you'll find in the next couple pages. It will give you the background you need to take control of your health.

Blood Sugar Control in Normal People

Most of your cells can run on several different kinds of fuel. One of them is a sugar called glucose. It is the sugar we refer to as **blood sugar**. Some glucose always circulates in the bloodstream, where it can be available to any cell that might need it. When you read that your blood sugar is 100 mg/dl, what this is really telling you is that there are 100 milligrams of glucose—one tenth of a gram, in every deciliter of your blood. A deciliter is one tenth of a liter. So if your blood sugar is 100 mg/dl you have 1 gram of glucose in every liter of blood.*

Everywhere except in the U.S., blood sugar is measured using a different measurement of concentration: mmol/L which stands for millimoles per liter. To convert mg/dl into mmol/L you divide mg/dl by 18.05. On Page 174 you will find a table you can use to find the mmol/L equivalent of any blood sugar mentioned in these pages.

Before most cells can use glucose, it must be transported inside the cells. Insulin is the hormone that makes this happen. That is why insulin is so important to blood sugar control. If there is no insulin available, no matter how much glucose is circulating in your bloodstream most of your cells will not be able to use it. And if the sugar in your blood isn't taken into cells, it will build up to dangerously high levels which will damage your organs and can even lead to death.

---

* All blood sugar meter readings discussed in this book are given as **plasma calibrated** values. Though all meters test only whole blood, plasma calibrated meters adjust the reading to match the value you'd get if you had your blood plasma tested at a lab. All meters currently sold in the U.S. use this kind of calibration. But some older meters and some meters sold in the UK are still **whole blood calibrated**. To convert a whole blood calibrated reading to a plasma calibrated reading, multiply it by 1.12. To convert the blood sugar measurements used here to whole blood calibrated values, divide by 1.12.

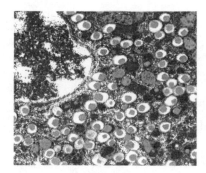

Figure 1. Beta cells in an Islet of Langerhans. The Beta cells in this picture are marked with gray dots

Insulin is produced by special cells called **beta cells**. These tiny cells are found in structures called the Islets of Langerhans which are scattered throughout your pancreas. The pancreas is an organ located near your liver that also secretes digestive enzymes. The job of the beta cell is to manufacture insulin, store it, and release it into the bloodstream when appropriate. Healthy beta cells are continually making insulin and storing it within the beta cell in the form of tiny granules.

The beta cells release this insulin into the bloodstream in two different ways. They release a continuous trickle of what is called **Basal Insulin** throughout the day and they also release larger bursts of insulin after you eat a meal. The meal time releases are called **First- and Second-Phase Insulin Release**.

Basal Insulin Release

The purpose of basal insulin release is to keep a small amount of insulin available in the bloodstream at all times. The beta cells of a healthy person release a small amount of insulin into the bloodstream in small pulses that occur every few minutes throughout the day and night. Maintaining this steady supply of insulin is important. It allows the cells of the body to utilize blood sugar whenever they need it.

During periods between meals the healthy beta cell also manufactures extra insulin and stores it in the form of granules for use at meal time. One of the things scientists have learned recently is that diabetes may develop when something disrupts the timing of this pulsed basal insulin release. Problems with basal insulin production can also keep the beta cells from storing the granules of insulin that will be used at meal times.

When you test your **fasting blood sugar** after not eating for eight hours or more, you are examining the health of your ability to secrete basal insulin. A normal or near normal fasting blood sugar means that your ability to secrete basal insulin is still intact. Truly normal fasting blood sugar values fall in the range between 70 and 85 mg/dl. Doctors will tell you that the normal range for a fasting blood sugar extends up to 100 mg/dl, but quite a lot of research has shown that people whose fasting blood sugar is over 90 mg/dl are very likely to develop diabetes within a decade, which suggests that it is not truly normal.

Insulin Levels Signal the Liver Whether More Glucose is Needed

The liver is the organ whose job is to add glucose to the blood stream if the blood sugar level starts to drop too low. If basal insulin production is working properly, the steady level of insulin in the bloodstream sends the signal to the liver that all is well and that no more glucose is needed. But if the insulin level drops during a fasting period, or if the liver becomes insulin resistant and does not respond to insulin signaling, the liver will assume that the glucose in the bloodstream is getting used up and more glucose is needed.

When the liver gets the signal that more glucose is needed, it turns to some carbohydrate it has stored for just this purpose. The term **carbohydrate** refers to the nutrients we call sugars and starches. The liver stores carbohydrate in the form of a substance called **glycogen**. To raise the blood sugar, the liver converts this glycogen into glucose and then dumps the resulting glucose into the bloodstream. This raises the blood sugar back to its normal level and ensures that cells will continue to have the fuel they need.

If it doesn't have enough glycogen stored, the liver can convert protein into glucose, too, and it will do this using protein from the food you have recently eaten. If you aren't eating enough protein, the body will break down the protein stored in your muscles, to provide the glucose the body needs.*

First-Phase Insulin Release

As soon as a healthy person starts to eat a meal, the parasympathetic nervous system sends out signals that begin the process that causes beta cells to release insulin into the bloodstream, beginning with the insulin they previously stored in granules.

As soon as the food hits the stomach, the carbohydrates in that food start to digest. Any pure glucose you have eaten goes immediately into the blood stream as it doesn't need to be broken down any further.

---

* This ability of the liver to turn muscle into glucose is why dieters lose muscle mass if they don't get enough protein when they are on stringent diets.

Fructose gets whisked away to your liver which converts it into fat. Digestive enzymes break down the rest of the carbohydrates in your meal into the two simple sugars, glucose and fructose, and that glucose goes into your bloodstream, too. It takes no more than 15 minutes after you have eaten a meal containing sugar or starch for the first glucose from the digested food to reach the bloodstream and begin raising the concentration of glucose in your blood.

Rising blood sugars now stimulate the beta cells to secrete more insulin. At the same time, as blood sugars rise to a threshold — somewhere between 100 and 120 mg/dl — **incretin hormones** released by the gut also stimulate the beta cells to secrete insulin. These early releases of insulin that occur as soon as you begin eating a meal are called **first-phase insulin release**. In a healthy person first-phase insulin release keeps the blood sugar from rising much over 125 mg/dl.

What cells take up that glucose? The brain and muscles have first dibs. Then the liver will use some glucose to top off its store of glycogen. But if your brain and muscle cells are all set for glucose and your liver has enough glycogen, insulin pushes glucose into *fat* cells. Insulin plays an important part in the process that transforms glucose into fat.

The amount of insulin a normal person's beta cells secrete during this first-phase insulin release is believed to be very close to the amount they needed to process the glucose produced by previous meals. If they usually eat a lot of carbohydrate, their body will release more insulin at the start of the next meal, even if that meal doesn't contain much carbohydrate. If this large dose of first-phase insulin doesn't meet up with enough incoming carbohydrate, it may drive the normal person's blood sugar low. When blood sugar drops too low, the brain senses it and sends out hunger signals that ramp up carbohydrate cravings. This is suggested as a reason why people with normal or near-normal metabolisms who have been eating a lot of carbohydrate may find themselves craving carbohydrates if they try to cut down on their carbohydrate intake.

If the normal person doesn't respond to the low blood sugar attack by eating more carbohydrate, their liver will transform stored glycogen into glucose and release that glucose into the blood stream until it has raised the blood sugar back to a normal level. When that person eats the next meal after the meal that resulted in a low blood sugar, their beta cells will release less first-phase insulin and avoid causing another low blood sugar.

In a healthy person, the first-phase insulin release peaks shortly after they've started their meal. The highest blood sugar level they will experience usually occurs by 45 minutes after they started eating.

Second-Phase Insulin Release

After completing this first-phase insulin release, the beta cells pause. But if the blood sugar is still not back under 100 mg/dl ten to twenty minutes later, beta cells start to secrete more insulin and provide another, smaller, **second-phase insulin release** whose job is to mop up the rest of the excess glucose circulating in the bloodstream. This second-phase insulin release continues as long as it is needed—until the blood sugar is back down to its fasting level. In a normal person, this usually takes about an hour to an hour and a half after the start of a meal.

It is this combination of a robust first-phase insulin release of stored insulin and a strong second-phase insulin release of secreted insulin that keeps the blood sugar of a normal person almost always under 100 mg/dl except for those few moments immediately after a meal before the first-phase insulin release kicks in. The system ensures that the brain and organs get a steady supply of glucose to fill their needs but prevents the build up of excess glucose in the blood stream that might clog up capillaries, gum up the kidneys, or inhibit the activity of nerves.

What are Truly Normal Blood Sugar Levels?

An illuminating research study presented by Professor J.S. Christiansen at the European Association for the Study of Diabetes conference in September of 2006 depicted the daily pattern of blood sugars in a group of normal subjects as it was revealed by the use of a **Continuous Glucose Monitoring System** (CGMS). The CGMS is a small computer attached to a probe. The probe is inserted under the skin where it samples the blood sugar every few minutes for a period lasting from a few days to several weeks. The computer stores and graphs this information.

Dr. Christiansen's data is summarized in Figure 2. A group of normal people wore the CGMS during the period spanning from when they woke up and ate breakfast until just before lunch. The heavy line shows the median blood sugar of the group as a whole. Next to it are thinner lines showing the top and bottom of the range within which most of their blood sugars fell. The lower set of lines represents their insulin and C-peptide levels.* The vertical line indicates the time when the study subjects ate a high carbohydrate breakfast.

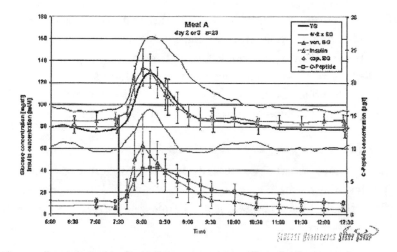

Figure 2. CGMS Study: Normal Blood Sugars

The data collected from these normal people showed that throughout the night their fasting blood glucose concentration remained flat in the low 80 mg/dl range. After a high carbohydrate meal, their blood sugar rose to a median value near 125 mg/dl for a brief period. This occurred about 45 minutes after they ate. In all but the people with the highest readings, blood sugar dropped back under 100 mg/dl by one hour and fifteen minutes after eating and it returned to 85 mg/dl by one hour and forty-five minutes after eating.

Note that even the highest of these normal readings is far below the cutoff most doctors consider to be the high end of "normal" which is 139 mg/dl measured *two hours after eating*!

---

* C-peptide is a byproduct of the manufacture of insulin. Measuring it is another way to measure insulin production.

Chapter Two
How Diabetes Develops

Now that you understand how the normal body controls blood sugar levels, it's time to look at what happens when that control breaks down. Before we do that, we need to take a moment to discuss the tests doctors and researchers use to measure blood sugar performance and to learn the terms doctors use to describe the various stages of deterioration that lie between normalcy and diabetes.

The Blood Sugar Tests Doctors Use

Table 1 shows the diagnostic criteria used to define normal blood sugar, the intermediate stage called "prediabetes," and diabetes.* The fasting criteria have changed several times, so current and historical ranges are both given.

Test	Normal	Prediabetes	Diabetes
Fasting Plasma Glucose (Current)	70-99	100 - 125	126+
Fasting Plasma Glucose (Before 1998)	70-110	110 – 139	140+
2-Hr OGTT (1978 – Today)	70 -139	140-199	200+

Table 1. Ranges for Diagnosing Blood Sugar Disorders, in mg/dl

Fasting Plasma Glucose

When researchers measure blood sugar they can choose from a couple different techniques. One is the **fasting plasma glucose** test, abbreviated **FPG**, a simple test which requires only a single blood draw. This test measures the concentration of glucose in the blood after an eight

---

* These criteria are set and periodically updated by a committee of experts appointed by the American Diabetes Association. Their choice of the specific cutoff points now in use is controversial and there is a lot of evidence that these criteria do not diagnose people until they have already had diabetes long enough to have developed diabetic complications that take years to emerge. You can read the details of how these criteria were chosen on **Bloodsugar101.com** at the subpage titled, **Misdiagnosis by Design**.

hour fast. The FPG only gives information about how the blood sugar behaves in the *fasting* state.

The American Diabetes Association has defined some arbitrary values which are used to determine if a person is normal, if they have an intermediate form of blood sugar dysfunction called **impaired fasting glucose (IFG)**, or if they have diabetes.

The ADA's definition of what fasting plasma glucose test values should be used for making these diagnoses has changed over the years. Until 1998 the ADA defined a fasting plasma glucose over 140 mg/dl as "diabetic." In 1998 they lowered the diabetes diagnostic cut-off to 126 mg/dl. The ADA has also lowered the value used to define the upward limit of "normal" several times. Its current value is 99 mg/dl.

This is why studies conducted before 1998 did not consider people to be diabetic unless their fasting blood sugars were over 140 mg/dl. Now that the diagnostic cutoff for the fasting plasma glucose test has dropped to 126 mg/dl, we know that a lot of people considered nondiabetic in older studies were actually diabetic, so some caution needs to be used when interpreting older studies.

The Oral Glucose Tolerance Test

The test used to track how first- and second-phase insulin release are holding up is the **Oral Glucose Tolerance Test** (OGTT). It is somewhat artificial in that it doesn't measure how people respond to food, but rather it measures how their blood sugar responds after consuming a huge dose of pure glucose. Glucose does not need to be digested, so it goes directly into the bloodstream almost as soon as you eat it. As a result, the OGTT is a brutal test which causes intense blood sugar swings that are much more severe than those you would experience eating the same amount of carbohydrate in the form of food.

The procedure for administering an OGTT is this: Subjects who have been fasting are given a fasting plasma glucose test. They then drink a glass containing 75 grams of glucose dissolved in water. After this, their blood sugar is measured at stated intervals, usually one hour and two hours after drinking the glucose. If a person's blood sugar is over 140 mg/dl two hours after drinking the glucose, the person is considered to have **prediabetes** or **impaired glucose tolerance (IGT)**. People whose blood sugar is under 140 mg/dl at two hours are considered to be normal, though there is no functional difference between what is happening in the body of the "normal" person whose blood sugar is 139 mg/dl two hours after drinking glucose and in that of the "prediabetic" person whose blood sugar at two hours is 140 mg/dl.

During the OGTT, if the blood sugar reading is higher than 199 mg/dl at two hours, the person is diagnosed as diabetic, not because there is any functional difference between a blood sugar that rises to 199 mg/dl and one that goes to 200 mg/dl, but simply because the ADA's Expert Panel arbitrarily chose this number as the level at which they would diagnose diabetes.

When discussing studies, any OGTT result cited is assumed to be a two hour result unless it is specifically described otherwise.

The A1c Test

The **A1c** test, which is also called the **Hemoglobin A_1c** test and abbreviated hgA_1c, is the test your doctor is most likely to rely on to track your blood sugar control over time. It is frequently used to measure blood sugar control in studies of large populations where it would be too expensive to perform individual glucose tolerance tests.

This test doesn't measure the concentration of sugar in your blood. Instead, it measures how much glucose has become permanently bonded to the hemoglobin in your red blood cells. The higher your blood sugar has been over an extended period of time, the more likely it is that glucose will have become permanently bonded to your hemoglobin. The A1c test result is expressed as a percentage since it reflects the percentage of red blood cells of a certain type that have glucose permanently bonded to them.

A normal A1c value is one between 4.0 and 5.0%. People with diabetes usually have A1cs ranging from 6.0% to as high as 15.0%.

Doctors use various formulas to compute the average blood sugar that they believe matches an A1c test result. The most commonly used formula is:

Average Blood Glucose = (A1c * 35.6) - 77.3

Because red blood cells usually live around three months, most doctors believe that the A1c reflects three months' worth of blood sugar control. However, studies suggest the A1c result largely reflects your blood sugar control in the two weeks before you took the test. Studies have also found that the height of post-meal blood sugar spikes greatly influences the A1c result in people with near normal blood sugars. The fasting blood sugar plays a larger part in raising the A1c when the A1c approaches 7.0%.

The A1c test will only reflect your average blood sugar control if you have a normal population of red blood cells. If you are anemic, by definition you have an abnormally low number of hemoglobin cells. This means you'll also have a deceptively low A1c reading, no matter how high your blood sugars have been in the period before the test.

Your A1c result may also be inaccurate if your red blood cells live longer or shorter than usual. Long-lived red blood cells can give a falsely high A1c reading because they continue to collect glucose during their longer lives. If your red blood cells are living shorter lives, they have less time to collect glucose. People with certain genetic variants of the red blood cell, including the sickle cell, also will get misleading A1c results.

The Patterns in Which Diabetes Develops

Now it's time to learn how normal blood sugar deteriorates into diabetes. We'll start out by looking at what two long-lasting studies of large populations have to teach us about the stages in which blood sugar control breaks down. Then we'll examine what is actually happening in your body during each of these stages.

A Landmark Study of Middle Aged People

Data from the Baltimore Longitudinal Study of Aging shows that over a period of ten years, the blood sugar of 48% of a large group of people in their 50s remained normal. Of the rest, 52% developed abnormal blood sugars, including the 11% who developed blood sugars bad enough to be diagnosed as diabetic.

By far the most prevalent pattern of blood sugar deterioration found in this group was the development of *impaired glucose tolerance with normal fasting blood sugar.* This means that their blood sugar was higher than 140 mg/dl two hours after consuming glucose but their fasting blood sugar remained under 110 mg/dl. It also probably implies that they were seeing blood sugars well over 140 mg/dl two hours after eating any meal containing carbohydrates.

Only 5% of the study subjects—one in twenty, developed the reverse pattern of impaired *fasting* glucose occuring with normal glucose

---

* The upper cutoff for normal fasting blood sugar used in this study was 110 mg/dl.

tolerance, while only 3% simultaneously developed both impaired glucose tolerance and impaired fasting glucose.

This makes it clear that it is far more common for *post-meal* blood sugar response to deteriorate before *fasting* blood sugar becomes impaired.

Outcome for 437 Originally Normal Subjects over a Decade of Observation Baltimore Longitudinal Study of Aging				
Nor-mal	IGT only	IGT and IFG	IFG only	Diabetes
48%	31%	3%	5%	11%

Table 2. Percentage of Middle Aged Subjects Developing Impaired Fasting Glucose (IFG), Impaired Glucose Tolerance (IGT), and Diabetes.

The Most Common Pattern for Those Developing Type 2 Diabetes

When the researchers turned their attention to the subset of people with abnormal blood sugars who had gone on to develop full-fledged diabetes, they found that, like the group as a whole, as they deteriorated they were much more likely to get abnormal two hour glucose tolerance test results while still having normal Fasting Plasma Glucose test results. Only a small number developed impaired fasting glucose while maintaining normal glucose tolerance.

This makes it very clear that deterioration of glucose tolerance—which implies deterioration in how blood sugar rises after a meal—is often the only apparent sign that a person is heading towards diabetes. For most people, the fasting blood sugar stays normal long after the meal-time control has faded out.

Of critical importance, in this study, *two thirds* of the people who were diagnosed as having diabetes using the glucose tolerance test had not yet developed impaired fasting glucose. Unfortunately, most doctors screen patients for diabetes using only the fasting blood sugar test since it is cheap and very easy to administer, unlike the time-consuming OGTT. Those doctors will not diagnose people who have become diabetic until much later in the deteriorative process.

This is why if you or a loved one are at risk for having diabetes you must insist that your doctor give you an OGTT. If that is not possible, buy a blood sugar meter and test your blood sugar after meals. That way you can learn if you have abnormal post-meal blood sugars early on, when you can still intervene and preserve your fasting blood sugar control and with it the lives of your remaining beta cells.

The Risk of Diabetes

The Baltimore Longitudinal Study of Aging diabetes study also found that a person in their fifties who has normal blood sugar has roughly a 1 in 8 chance of becoming diabetic over the next decade. A person who already has impaired glucose tolerance has a 4 in 10 chance of progressing to diabetes over a decade while a person with impaired fasting glucose has almost a 1 in 2 chance of progressing to diabetes. Again, this suggests that fasting blood sugar control is the last part of blood sugar control to deteriorate.

Who Progresses?

The Baltimore Longitudinal Study of Aging data gives us some further insight into who develops diabetes in which pattern.

When analyzing data about the people who progressed to full-fledged diabetes, the researchers found that people older than 56 years were more likely to first develop impaired glucose tolerance than were younger people. The risk of developing impaired fasting glucose was about the same for all age groups.

They also found that men were more likely to see a deterioration in their fasting glucose than women, as were subjects with overall or central obesity when compared with lean subjects.

A Second Study Finds Diabetes Does Not Develop Gradually

Another interesting study conducted in a large population looked at how the blood sugar of the *individuals* in that study changed over time.

The researchers studied a population of people living in Mexico City who were deemed to be at risk for diabetes. Every three years they measured the subjects' fasting plasma glucose and their fasting insulin levels. They also administered oral glucose tolerance tests.

The researchers in this second study found that rather than being a gradual process, the transition to diabetes appeared to occur very quickly within a single three year period and that it was characterized by a sudden and very swift increase in fasting glucose values.

A Swift and Unexpected Deterioration in Blood Sugar Control Precedes the Diagnosis of Diabetes

One in twelve of the study subjects went from having normal glucose tolerance to having full-fledged diabetes during the three years between one examination and the next. Slightly fewer—One in fourteen—went from having impaired glucose tolerance to diabetes over the same three year period.

While the fasting plasma glucose of those who did *not* become diabetic increased "slightly and in an apparently linear manner," that of the people who became diabetic took a sudden step up, showing an average gain of 50 mg/dl between one examination and the next, three years later. The two hour oral glucose tolerance test results showed a similar pattern. The people who did *not* become diabetic showed a "slight increase" in their blood sugar values on the OGTT over the three year period while those who became diabetic saw an average surge of 108 mg/dl between one exam and the next, three years later.

That this change was very sudden was highlighted by the discovery that the people who became diabetic during one three year period had shown very little change in their blood sugars over the three year period *before* the one in which their blood sugar deteriorated so swiftly. In fact, the changes in their blood sugar in that earlier period were the same as those in people who stayed normal.

This sudden and rapid deterioration after a period where blood sugar response stays relatively constant may happen when the post-meal blood sugar level finally rises above the threshold where insulin resistance suddenly increases dramatically and where glucose toxicity starts to poison beta cells.

What this study didn't discover, but many of us active on the Web have found to be true, is that just as blood sugar control appears to deteriorate dramatically when you hit a certain high blood sugar threshold, when you take the steps needed to bring your post-meal blood sugars down below that critical level, you will often see a similarly dramatic rate of improvement.

What Happens at Each Stage of Breakdown?

Prediabetes

Remember the two stages of post-meal insulin release we described in Chapter One: The first-phase release of insulin that was previously stored in granules and the second-phase release of insulin secreted in real-time by your beta cells? Well, for most people, the first stage in the breakdown of blood sugar control happens when the first-phase insulin release after a meal stops working properly.

When you don't get a swift release of stored insulin as soon as you start to eat a meal containing carbohydrates, your blood sugar will rise much higher than a normal 125 mg/dl. Now all you can rely on to lower your post-meal blood sugar is the slower, weaker second-phase insulin release that only kicks in about a half hour after you start eating. This second-phase insulin release is slow because it requires your beta cells to secrete insulin rather than use the insulin they previously stored. Now rather than peaking no more than 45 minutes after eating, the highest blood sugar you see after a meal will occur at least an hour after eating, possibly later. After it peaks, it may take another hour or longer for your blood sugar to return to normal.

This is clearly no longer normal. But it is not until the blood sugar remains above 139 mg/dl two hours after eating that doctors will diagnose **prediabetes** which is also known as **impaired glucose tolerance (IGT)**. A diagnosis of prediabetes is a very strong sign that your first-phase insulin release has been failing for a while and that you are now relying on second-phase insulin release to return your post-meal blood sugars to a normal level.

Many people remain prediabetic for the rest of their life and never progress to diabetes. Even so, they may develop what doctors consider to be diabetic complications. This is because when you rely on your second-phase insulin release to control your blood sugar level after eating, it may take as many as three to five hours for your blood sugar level to return to normal. Since you eat every couple hours during the day, you will rarely get back to a normal blood sugar level between meals. This is a huge problem, because, as you will see in Chapter Four, scientists are discovering that it is hours of exposure to blood sugars in the so-called *prediabetic* range that cause *diabetic* complications.

Diabetes

The American Diabetes Association defines several different criteria for diagnosing diabetes. One states that a person should be diagnosed with diabetes when a random blood test reveals a blood sugar level higher than 200 mg/dl. By the time this has happened, you have usually lost all of your first-phase insulin release and are relying on a weakened second-phase insulin release to bring your blood sugars back down after eating. If you continue to let your blood sugars rise very high after meals, eventually your second-phase insulin release will fade out too, and you will end up with blood sugars that spend most of their time at the extremely high blood sugars characteristic of people diagnosed with diabetes—blood sugars that range from 200 to 500 mg/dl.

When both first- and second-phase insulin release fail after meals, your fasting blood sugar usually starts to skyrocket, too.

Impaired Fasting Glucose

There's some evidence that for most of us it is the strain of coping with the loss of the first-phase insulin release that raises our fasting blood sugar. This is because when your post-meal blood sugars reach the diabetic range and your second-phase insulin release grows weaker, it may take four or five hours for your beta cells to secrete enough insulin to bring your blood sugar level down to its fasting level. In fact, during the day your blood sugar may never get back to a normal fasting level because glucose coming in from your next meal enters the bloodstream before glucose from the previous meal has been completely cleared. Only at night, while you are sleeping, will your beta cells finally be able to secrete enough insulin to lower your blood sugar enough to give you a normal fasting blood sugar.

However, since it took all the insulin your beta cells could make to lower you blood sugar to a normal level, your beta cells have had no chance to store any extra insulin to take care of your breakfast. As soon as you eat a bowl of cereal, your blood glucose will start to rise again. With no stored insulin to draw on, your beta cells will once again have to spend many hours lowering your blood sugar.

Eventually, even the long hours of the night will not be enough time for your beta cells to produce the insulin you need to bring your blood sugar back to normal. Only then, perhaps a decade after you developed diabetic *post-meal* blood sugar readings, will you finally start seeing diabetic *fasting* blood sugar levels.

This process explains why, for most people who become diabetic, the fasting blood sugar level is the very last measurement to become abnormal. Only when your beta cells can't bring your blood sugar down to near-normal levels after eight long hours will you be diagnosed as diabetic by a doctor who relies on the fasting blood sugar test. Unfortunately, it is this fasting blood sugar test alone that most doctors use to screen for diabetes. This means you may actually have had diabetes for up to a decade before your doctor gives you a formal diagnosis.

Why Insulin Release Fails

Insulin Resistance

First- and second-phase insulin releases may fail to do their jobs for several reasons. The most common is the condition called **insulin resistance** in which receptors in the liver and the muscle cells stop responding properly to insulin. If high blood sugars are due solely to insulin resistance there may be a lot of insulin circulating in the body, but insulin resistant muscles or an insulin resistant liver don't respond to that insulin until its level rises abnormally high.

When a person's cells become insulin resistant, it takes a lot more insulin than normal to push circulating glucose into cells. In this case, while a person might have a perfectly normal first- and second-phase insulin release, the first-phase release might not produce enough insulin to clear the circulating blood glucose that results from eating a high carbohydrate meal.

The second-phase release might be prolonged in an insulin resistant person because it takes a long time for beta cells to secrete the large amount of insulin needed to counter the insulin resistance. Eventually the body may not be able to produce enough insulin to clear all the dietary carbohydrate from the bloodstream, and blood sugars will remain at abnormal levels all the time.

If insulin resistance at the muscles and liver is your only problem and you have not inherited diabetic genes, over time you may be able to grow new pancreas islets filled with new beta cells that can secrete and store the huge amounts of insulin you need to use for your first- and second-phase insulin release. This is what happens to a lot of obese people who are often very insulin resistant but never become diabetic.

It is precisely because most people *can* grow new beta cells, even when their blood sugar rises into the prediabetic range that many people with prediabetes don't deteriorate past the pre-diabetic stage to full-fledged diabetes. Even so, they may be diagnosed with "Metabolic

Syndrome" and develop obesity, high blood pressure, and a higher risk of having a heart attack. All of these are probably side effects of the very high levels of insulin their bodies are producing. But these people do not go on to develop the extremely high blood sugars characteristic of diabetes. Recent epidemiological studies have estimated the prevalence of metabolic syndrome in the U.S. at 23% while the prevalence of Type 2 Diabetes is only 8%.

You may infer that insulin resistance is playing some role in your own case if you have been battling weight gain and have found it impossible to lose weight on a low fat diet.* This is because, unlike muscle cells, fat cells do not become insulin resistant, so the high levels of circulating insulin characteristic of insulin resistance push glucose into fat cells and cause weight gain, especially in the abdominal area, as the fat stored there is most sensitive to insulin.

Unfortunately, when you have impaired glucose tolerance, there is no sure way of knowing for certain if your rising blood sugars are due solely to insulin resistance or to a more worrisome cause: failing beta cells.

Failing Beta Cells

Insulin release also fails when beta cells lose their ability to secrete insulin. This can happen along with insulin resistance or without it. Studies have found that young, thin, non-insulin resistant relatives of insulin resistant people who have Type 2 Diabetes already show signs of beta cell dysfunction that is probably of genetic origin. As we mentioned earlier, a slow autoimmune attack can kill off your beta cells and limit your ability to secrete insulin.

If your beta cells aren't working properly, you are more likely to develop full-fledged diabetes. Your damaged beta cells will have to work full-time just to keep up with the need for a basal insulin release. This keeps them from storing any excess in granules for later release.

One intriguing study suggests that some people with Type 2 Diabetes may have a defect which makes their beta cells die when these cells attempt to reproduce. If these people become insulin resistant, the need for more insulin may cause their beta cells to try to divide and then die, hastening the degenerative process.

---

* Research shows that people who are not insulin resistant can lose weight equally well on any type of diet, while people who are insulin resistant will lose weight more easily on a low carbohydrate diet that reduces their level of circulating insulin.

Other people whose beta cells are failing may have a recently discovered slow-developing form of autoimmune diabetes called **LADA** (Latent Autoimmune Diabetes of Adults) where beta cells die gradually rather than all at once, as they do in Type 1 Diabetes, the more familiar form of autoimmune diabetes that is usually diagnosed in children. We'll discuss LADA later in Chapter Twelve.

Infections, toxic chemicals, pesticides, and some pharmaceutical drugs can also kill or cripple beta cells. And though it is a rare cause for diabetic blood sugars, pancreatic tumors can also cause beta cells to stop secreting insulin.

Rising Blood Sugars Further Damage Beta Cells

Whatever the reason for your failing insulin releases there's an ugly feedback mechanism that kicks in as your blood sugar rises after meals. High blood sugar itself is toxic to beta cells, a phenomenon called **glucose toxicity**. So as your blood sugar rises, for whatever reason, it causes further damage to your beta cells, which makes your second-phase insulin release even less able to lower your blood sugar.

Rising Blood Sugars Increase Insulin Resistance

When your blood sugar is routinely going over 180 mg/dl, another bad thing happens. Your cells become insulin resistant *even if they weren't insulin resistant before.* So now it takes even more insulin to lower your blood sugar. The reason for this is that the gene that regulates insulin resistance in muscles is shut off by high blood sugar levels. Fortunately, this gene will start working again when blood sugars are lowered.

The Fasting Blood Sugar Death Spiral

When the beta cells are no longer able to secrete enough insulin to keep fasting blood sugar normal, it often means you have suffered a critical amount of irreversible beta cell death.When this happens, blood sugar control can deteriorate very swiftly. Remember how we explained earlier that the liver interprets a low insulin level as a sign that blood sugar is low? When the beta cells no longer provide a steady basal insulin release, the liver takes it as a sign that blood sugar is low and then, no matter how high your blood sugar might be, the liver dumps more glucose into your bloodstream.

This effect may explain why fasting blood sugar tends not to deteriorate slowly and steadily but often takes a sudden upward surge of

50 mg/dl or more around the time a person has become diabetic enough for a doctor to notice it and give a diagnosis.

A Different Syndrome: Impaired Fasting Glucose with Normal Post-Meal Control

As we saw when we looked at the Baltimore Longitudinal Study of Aging data, there is a very small subset of people, mostly men, whose *fasting blood sugar* rises quite high, perhaps even into the diabetic range, while their post-meal blood sugars remain normal or near normal. They appear to have a different syndrome than the majority, whose post-meal blood sugars deteriorate first. Scientists speculate that these people may have a defect that affects only their ability to secrete basal insulin.

How Many Beta Cells Have to Die to Ruin Blood Sugar Control?

This question was answered by a series of autopsies a team of researchers performed on pancreases taken from Mayo Clinic patients whose medical histories were known. They found that the pancreases of obese patients who had had normal blood sugars had 50% *more* beta cells than non-obese normal people. This demonstrated that they had been able to grow new beta cells when they were needed. In contrast, obese patients who had had fasting blood sugars that had risen into the prediabetic impaired range had lost about 40% of their beta cell mass. Patients diagnosed with fully diabetic fasting blood sugars had 63% less beta cell mass than normal people—which the researchers attributed to beta cell death, not to any shrinking in the size of the beta cells. There was more evidence of recent beta cell death in lean people with diabetes than in obese people with diabetes.

But this is not entirely bad news, as it tells us that even after a diagnosis of prediabetes or diabetes, most people—especially those who are obese—still have a significant amount of beta cells remaining. This is the main *functional* difference between Type 2 Diabetes and Type 1 Diabetes. People with Type 1 Diabetes usually have lost *all* their beta cells due to an autoimmune attack.

And when you have living beta cells left, it is a lot easier to regain control than when you don't, because there are effective strategies you can use take the strain off those remaining beta cells and help them do their job.

Chapter Three
What Really Causes Diabetes?

Get Rid of the Guilt!

Before we discuss how you can normalize your broken blood sugar metabolism, there's something we need to get straight.

You did not cause your diabetes through reckless overeating and criminal laziness.

Despite everything you have read in the media, and contrary to what your doctor may have told you, diabetes is *not* caused by obesity. You did not give yourself diabetes thanks to gluttony and sloth.

Because the media have publicized the toxic myth that people with diabetes are responsible for their plight, we're going to take a few moments now to examine what scientists have learned about the real relationship between diabetes and obesity and why *it is much more likely that your diabetes caused your obesity than the other way around.*

A Toxic Myth That Harms People with Diabetes

You have probably already been brutalized by the many statements that appear in the media to the effect that people with diabetes are diabetic because they are lazy gluttons.

These statements might have motivated you to ignore early warning signs that your blood sugar was not normal. If so, you are not alone. The fear of being labeled a self-destructive glutton frightens many people into avoiding the early diabetes diagnosis that could completely eliminate all diabetic complications.

Once you were diagnosed, these media pronouncements may have filled you with self-hatred that made it all the more difficult to cope with your new diagnosis The belief that faulty behavior caused your diabetes leads to depression, self-loathing, and feelings of helplessness. If you think you are a rotten slob whose moral weakness gave you this crummy disease, you aren't likely to believe you have the ability to prevent further decline.

Even worse, the belief that people with diabetes have brought their disease on themselves inclines doctors to assume that since their diabetic patients did nothing to prevent their disease, they won't make the effort to control it — a belief that may lead to them to give people with diabetes mediocre care — which is precisely the kind of care most surveys show doctors give to people with diabetes — care that ensures people with diabetes will end up with the tragic complications that shorten their lives and fill their declining years with suffering.

The myth that diabetes is caused by overeating also hurts the one out of five people with Type 2 Diabetes who are *not* overweight. Because doctors only think "Diabetes" when they see a patient who fits the stereotype — the obese, sedentary patient — they often neglect to check people of normal weight for blood sugar disorders, even when they show up with such classic symptoms of high blood sugar as recurrent urinary tract infections, fungal complaints, or neuropathy.

Where Did This Toxic Myth Come From?

Because most people who are obese are insulin resistant — including the two thirds of obese people who do not ever develop diabetes — the conclusion was drawn years ago that the insulin resistance seen in people with Type 2 Diabetes was caused by their obesity. It made sense. Something was burning out the beta cells in these people, and it seemed logical that it must be the stress of pumping out huge amounts of insulin, day after day, to meet the needs of the obese, insulin resistant body.

Some studies also showed that substances secreted by fat cells seemed to increase insulin resistance. This, reinforced the idea that the insulin resistance seen in people with Type 2 diabetes was caused by their obesity.

This is why it is common for doctors to tell a patient who has just been diagnosed with diabetes that their diabetes was caused by their obesity and that if they could lose as little as ten pounds they would no longer be diabetic. Though as any person with diabetes who has lost ten pounds — or even fifty pounds — can tell you, this is almost never true.

But doctors who believe that diabetes could be easily reversed if people would only stop stuffing themselves with food often feel about people with diabetes much the way they do about those smokers who refuse to stop smoking even after they develop lung cancer. They may secretly feel contempt for the fat person with diabetes who shows up in their office and wish they'd go away and do their self-induced deteriorating somewhere decent people don't have to watch them.

With an attitude like this, it's no surprise that many doctors don't keep up on diabetes research. They don't take seminars about the latest ways to treat diabetes. They save their energy to treat patients they think of as more deserving and because they are ignorant about the real causes of diabetes they reinforce the self-hatred of their patients with diabetes and do not challenge the media when they spread misinformation suggesting that diabetes is the punishment fat people bring on themselves for being lazy gluttons.

Though it is completely not true.

Proof that Obesity Doesn't Cause Diabetes

While people who have diabetes are often heavy, one out of five people diagnosed with Type 2 Diabetes is thin or of normal weight. And though heavy people with Type 2 Diabetes *are* likely to be insulin resistant, the majority of insulin resistant obese people will *never* develop diabetes even though they are just as insulin resistant as those who do.

The message that diabetes researchers in academic laboratories are coming up with is quite different from what you read in the media. They are finding that to develop diabetes, you need to have at least one of many different metabolic flaws. Most of these flaws appear to be genetic in origin. Some are inherited, but others are caused by exposure to chemical toxins.

Unless you have damaged genes, you can eat until you drop and though you may get very fat and develop quite a few other health problems, your blood sugar control will stay functional and you will *never* develop diabetes.

Twin Studies Back Up a Genetic Cause for Diabetes

Studies of identical twins showed that twins have an 80% concordance for Type 2 Diabetes. In other words, if one twin has Type 2 Diabetes, the chances that the other twin will also get it are four out of five. While some might argue that this could be explained by the fact that identical twins were raised in the same home by the same mother who fed them the same unhealthy diet, studies of fraternal twins found *no* such concordance. Even when they are raised by the same caregivers and fed the same diet, there is a much lower likelihood that two fraternal twins will develop diabetes.

These findings begin to hint that diabetes is caused by more than bad habits. Identical twins have identical genes. Non-identical, fraternal twins do not. When identical twins share a trait much more frequently than do fraternal twins, scientists suspect a genetic cause for that trait.

Scientists have been hard at work searching for the genes that interfere with the normal mechanisms the body uses to regulate blood sugar. The genes they have so far come up with that are thought to cause Type 2 Diabetes include TCF7L2, HNF4-a, PTPN, SHIP2, and ENPP1. There are many more. New diabetes genes are being discovered every year.

Since twin studies show that both identical twins do not *always* develop diabetes, this tells scientists that additional factors beyond the presence of an inherited gene must be needed to produce diabetes. Scientists call these **environmental factors**. Quite a few studies hint at what environmental factors might cause a person carrying a borderline gene to develop full-fledged diabetes.

A Mother's Diet During Pregnancy May Cause Diabetes

Researchers following the children of mothers who had experienced a Dutch famine during World War II found that children of mothers who had experienced famine were far more likely to develop diabetes in later life than a control group from the same population whose mothers had been adequately fed.

This may not seem all that relevant to Americans whose mothers have not been exposed to famine conditions. But to conclude this is to forget how many American teens and young women suffer from eating disorders and how prevalent crash dieting is in the group of women most likely to get pregnant.

It is also significant that until the 1980s obstetricians routinely warned pregnant women against gaining what is now understood to be a healthy amount of weight. When pregnant women started to gain weight, doctors often put them on highly restrictive diets which resulted in their giving birth to underweight babies whose low birth weight suggests that they were starved in the womb.

A Mother's Gestational Diabetes May Cause Diabetes

Maternal starvation is not the only pre-birth factor associated with an increased risk of diabetes. Several studies have shown that having a well-fed mother who suffered gestational diabetes also increases a child's risk of developing diabetes.

A child who inherits a known diabetes gene from their mother is more likely to express that gene more severely than if they inherit the identical gene from their father — probably because a mother carrying a diabetes gene will have a diabetic pregnancy.

Insulin Resistance is Found in Thin Relatives of People with Type 2 Diabetes

Lab research has come up with some intriguing findings that challenge the idea that obesity causes insulin resistance and that in turn causes Type 2 diabetes.

One of these studies took two groups of *thin* subjects with normal blood sugar who were evenly matched for height and weight. The two groups differed only in that one group had close relatives who had developed Type 2 Diabetes, and hence, if there were a genetic component to Type 2 Diabetes, they were more likely to have it. The other group had no relatives with Type 2 Diabetes.

The researchers measured the subjects' insulin resistance and discovered that the thin relatives of the people with Type 2 Diabetes already had much more insulin resistance than did the thin people identical to them in height and weight who had no relatives with diabetes.

Mitochondrial Dysfunction is Found in Lean Relatives of People with Type 2 Diabetes

Why this might be was made clear by a landmark 2004 study which looked at the cells of some of these "healthy, young, lean" but insulin-resistant relatives of people with Type 2 Diabetes.

The study found that in thin people who had relatives with Type 2 Diabetes, the mitochondria, which are the parts of the cell that actually burn glucose, appeared to have a defect. While the mitochondria of people who had no relatives with diabetes burned glucose well, the mitochondria of the people with an inherited genetic predisposition to diabetes were not able to burn off glucose as efficiently. Not only that, but this mitochondrial flaw caused the glucose they could not burn to be stored in their cells as fat.

More Evidence that Abnormal Insulin Resistance Precedes Weight Gain and Probably Causes it

A study that used a new imaging technology compared the energy usage of lean people who were insulin resistant with that of lean people who were insulin sensitive. These researchers found that lean but insulin resistant subjects converted the glucose that came from high carbohydrate meals into triglycerides—i.e. fat. In contrast, lean insulin-sensitive subjects stored that same glucose in the form of glycogen—the storage form of carbohydrate found in muscles and the liver.

The researchers concluded that "the insulin resistance, in these young, lean, insulin resistant individuals, was independent of abdominal obesity and circulating plasma adipocytokines, suggesting that these abnormalities develop later in the development of the metabolic syndrome."

Translated into English, what this means is that *people become insulin resistant before they become fat.* More importantly, their insulin resistance clearly had not been caused by the chemicals given off by fat cells, because they didn't have these fat-related chemicals in their bloodstreams. Or to put it another way, these researchers concluded that obesity was the result, not the cause, of the metabolic flaw that led these people to store glucose from high carbohydrate meals as fat rather than in the form of easy-to-burn glycogen, as people not fated to develop diabetes would have done.

Beta Cells Fail to Reproduce in People with Diabetes

The study of pancreas autopsies cited earlier found that fat, insulin-resistant people who did not develop diabetes apparently were able to grow new beta cells to produce the extra insulin they needed. They had 50% more beta cells than did people of normal weight without blood sugar problems. In contrast, the beta cells of people who developed diabetes were unable to reproduce.

Autoimmune Diabetes "Indistinguishable" from Type 2 Diabetes

Though doctors have for years made a clear distinction between people with autoimmune Type 1 Diabetes—which they believed was not their fault—and those with Type 2 Diabetes—which *was,* a study published in the journal *Diabetes Care* in April of 2007 found that fully 4.5% of a sample of 4,250 people diagnosed as "Type 2" diabetics had the kind of antibodies which are the diagnostic sign of autoimmune diabetes. The researcher who discovered this noted that slowly progressive autoimmune diabetes in adults is often indistinguishable from classic Type 2 Diabetes.

Autoimmune diabetes is caused when the body's own immune system confuses the beta cell with a disease-causing invader and attacks it. If the attack is robust, most of the beta cells die and the person ends up with Type 1 diabetes. However, the finding of this new study suggests that some people get a "mild" autoimmune attack that kills off just enough beta cells to cause a mild form of autoimmune diabetes that is easily confused with Type 2—especially if it happens to someone over age twenty. Autoimmune diabetes is even more likely to be misdiagnosed if a person is at all overweight—as a large proportion of the entire population now is.

To further complicate matters, people with autoimmune thyroid disease or autoimmune arthritis may become obese because of the drugs they have to take, so when they get a second autoimmune disease—diabetes—their obesity may cause their doctors to make an incorrect diagnosis.

Pesticides and PCBs in the Bloodstream Correlate with the Incidence of Diabetes Independent of Weight

A more chilling finding is this: A study conducted among members of New York State's Mohawk tribe found that the odds of being diagnosed with diabetes in this population were almost four times higher than normal in members who had high concentrations of PCBs in their blood serum. Even worse was the incidence of diabetes in those with high concentrations of pesticides in their blood. This relationship held true regardless of their weight. There is no reason to believe this phenomenon is limited to people of Native American heritage. For generations, the entire population of the U.S. has been overexposed to powerful pesticides.

Plastics in Most Humans' Bloodstreams May Cause Diabetes

A CDC study published in 2007 found that 92% of 2,500 people studied had detectable amounts of Bisphenol-A in their urine. Bisphenol-A is a plastic used in the water bottle you take to the gym and the baby bottle you give your infant. It has been shown in animal studies to significantly diminish insulin sensitivity.

An article that discusses some disturbing results of animal research that linked exposure to Bisphenol-A to obesity and diabetes includes the revealing photo you see in Figure 3. The mouse on the right is normal. The other was exposed to Bisphenol-A in the womb and sustained genetic damage. It looks like a lot of folks you see strolling through the mall.

Another recent study reports that heating a plastic baby bottle releases surprising amounts of Bisphenol-A. When the bottle's contents are drunk, it results in a concentration of the chemical in human blood that is far higher than the level known to cause harm.

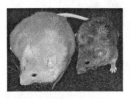

Can it be coincidental that the huge increase in obesity and diabetes seems to have begun shortly after plastics began to replace glass, metal, wood, and cellulose-based products in our environment?

Figure 3. Mouse on left exposed to Bisphenol-A in womb

Prescription Drugs Cause Both Obesity and Diabetes

The media never mentions this, but many commonly prescribed drugs also are known to cause diabetes. Beta blockers prescribed for blood pressure control and atypical antipsychotic drugs like Zyprexa have been shown to cause diabetes in people who would not otherwise get it. Prednisone and other corticosteroids increase insulin resistance and may permanently worsen blood sugar in people whose blood sugar control was marginal before starting on cortisone therapy. Other drugs that can cause diabetes include some drugs used in chemotherapy and anti-rejection drugs used after organ transplants.

Research suggests that SSRI antidepressants can exacerbate insulin resistance. It is well known that several SSRI antidepressants cause weight gain. Some studies suggest that people taking SSRIs are also more likely to develop diabetes.

The drug companies that earn huge profits from selling antidepressants argue that depression is a side effect of the underlying condition that eventually turns into Type 2 Diabetes and that people who develop diabetes while taking SSRIs must have already had abnormal blood sugars before they started them. But this is by no means clear. Other psychiatric drugs, most notoriously Zyprexa, are well-known to cause diabetes in people who started out with completely normal blood sugars.

A New Model for How Diabetes Develops

These research findings open up a new way of understanding the relationship between obesity and diabetes.

Perhaps people start out with genetic conditions which make them insulin resistant even when young and thin and cause their bodies to store carbohydrate as fat in situations where a normal person would burn it or store it as glycogen. Perhaps they start out genetically normal, but become insulin resistant thanks to exposure to a pesticide or the Bisphenol-A that leached out of their baby bottles. Or perhaps they were given a prescription medication that made them much more insulin resistant than normal.

Now consider what happens if that person who has become insulin resistant for whatever reason *also* has some condition which makes their beta cells unable to reproduce normally — as has been observed to be the case with people who have diabetes. Put this all together and you suddenly get a fatal combination that is almost guaranteed to make a person fat.

Insulin resistance leads to rising blood sugars. These damage beta cells. In a normal person who has the ability to grow new beta cells, any damaged beta cells will be supplemented by new ones which keeps their blood sugar low enough to avoid further damage. But the beta cells of a person with the kinds of damage we're discussing are unable to reproduce. Once their blood sugar starts to rise, more beta cells succumb to the glucose toxicity. That, in turn, raises their blood sugar higher.

As the concentration of glucose in their blood rises, these people are not able to do what a normal person does with excess blood sugar — which is to burn it for energy. Instead their defective mitochondria will cause the excess glucose to be stored as fat. As this fat gets stored in their muscles it causes even more insulin resistance — long before the individual begins to gain visible weight.

Then it is only a matter of time until accumulating fat stores start secreting substances known to further worsen insulin resistance. It takes more and more insulin to lower their rising blood sugars. We know that although high levels of insulin may not lower blood sugars effectively in people who are insulin resistant, that insulin still pushes glucose into their fat cells which don't become insulin resistant the way muscle cells do.

Eventually the person becomes visibly fat. Their rising blood sugars make their insulin resistance even worse. When those high blood sugars have killed off 60% of their beta cells, their fasting blood sugar finally rises, and the person, by now obese and highly insulin resistant, ends up, at last, with a diabetes diagnosis.

Low Fat Diets Promote the Deterioration that Leads to Diabetes in People with the Genetic Predisposition

In the past two decades, when people who were heading towards diabetes began to gain weight they were advised to eat a low fat diet. Unfortunately, this low fat diet is also a high carbohydrate diet—one that exacerbates blood sugar problems. The high carbohydrate content of low fat diets raises blood sugars dangerously high after each meal.

So as people who were prediabetic attempted to diet off the weight that was starting to accumulate, their low fat diets worsened their blood sugars, speeding them to the point where their post-meal blood sugars were so high that they greatly increased the person's insulin resistance. Their increasing insulin resistance promoted even more fat storage, and the diet failed. If you have ever eaten a low fat diet consisting of only a carefully counted 1,200 calories per day, every day for a month, and lost no weight at all, as I did, you know what I'm talking about. After failing to losing weight time after time, most rational people will give up on dieting. This is1 exactly what many people with diabetes reported happened to them.

The Relentless Hunger Caused by Deteriorating Blood Sugars Leads to Dramatic Weight Gain

If you believe that, despite what you just read, it was your own out-of-control eating that caused your diabetes, you may be relieved to know that it is very likely that it was nothing else but undiagnosed diabetic high blood sugars that caused your gluttony.

Long before a person develops diabetes, they go through that phase where first-phase insulin secretion has failed and blood sugars rise into the prediabetic range after every meal. Every time they eat a meal containing carbohydrates, their blood sugar rockets up and stays high for an hour or two before the lagging second-phase insulin release finally puts out enough insulin to drop it back to a normal level.

In this prediabetic state, the beta cells are pumping out insulin as fast as their little membranes can manage it and they often put out *too much* insulin. So instead of returning to a normal fasting level, the blood sugar may plunge to a *low*. This phenomenon is often called **reactive hypoglycemia**.

What many people don't realize is that when your blood sugar drops swiftly you may experience intense hunger. The reasons for this are not completely clear, but may have to do with your brain's fear that the blood sugar may drop so low as to endanger consciousness. Though this is unlikely to occur, your brain believes it will, so it floods you with the feeling that if you don't eat some carbohydrates — now — you are going to die.

The intense hunger caused by blood sugar swings can develop years before your blood sugar reaches the level where you will be diagnosed as diabetic. The higher your blood sugars go, the more intense the hunger you feel as they drop back down. This is why, as your blood sugar control deteriorated, you may have found yourself hungrier after eating a high carbohydrate meal than you were before you started. And that hunger may have compelled you to eat more and more, until you really were completely out of control.

The problem is not moral, it is physiological. But this kind of relentless hunger is often the very first diabetic symptom a person will experience. It can make you eat with a terrifying ravenousness that can make you feel depraved. You aren't. You're experiencing blood sugar swings. It's a known problem with a known cure, but sadly, most doctors do not recognize this kind of hunger as a symptom. Indeed, if you tell your doctor you are experiencing overwhelming hunger, he is likely to suggest that you have an emotional problem and give you an antidepressant — which will worsen your insulin resistance! If you are a middle aged female, doctors may blame your sudden and terrifying weight gain on menopausal changes.

But here's the good news. Once you know that you have a blood sugar abnormality, be it prediabetes or full blown diabetes, your days of misery, hunger, and out of control eating are over. Not because you are going to turn into a better person and rediscover some hidden source of will power, but because there are well understood ways of dealing with a broken blood sugar metabolism that eliminate the hunger, reduce the insulin resistance, and free you from the domination of blood sugar swings.

And you don't have to lose a single pound make it happen!

Chapter Four
Blood Sugar Level and Organ Damage

Now that you know you have abnormally high blood sugars the obvious question is this: What blood sugar levels cause the terrible organ damage doctors describe with the euphemism "diabetic complications"?

Surprisingly, there is very little medical research directed at answering this question. Almost all the diabetes-related research you see reported in the medical news is research about the benefits of this or that new drug. Since none of the diabetic drugs lower blood sugar very much, these studies are careful to avoid connecting the blood sugar levels the drugs make possible with the incidence of complications that develop in the people who take those drugs.

The studies that connect blood sugar levels to organ damage rarely make their way into the medical press. To find them, you must comb through obscure research studies published by academic researchers. But the information is there. Taken together, quite a few studies performed by scientists from many different disciplines using many different research techniques all seem to point to a narrow range of blood sugars as being where the various diabetic complications begin.

In this chapter, we'll summarize what these somewhat obscure studies tell us about what blood sugar levels bring about organ damage. If you want to read the actual research papers, you'll find the citations in the Reference section on Page 183. You will find links to those studies at **Bloodsugar101.com** as well as new studies published since this book was published.

Blood Sugar Level and Nerve Damage

Neuropathy appears to strike when blood sugars remain over 140 mg/dl for two hours or more. **Neuropathy** is a word which means "sick nerves," and nerve damage is one of the earliest and most devastating diabetic complications.

Because nerves start to become damaged at the "mildly" elevated blood sugar level most doctors ignore, almost one half of people with

Type 2 Diabetes already have detectable neuropathy by the time they are diagnosed with diabetes. Many other people who are *never* officially diagnosed with diabetes but have higher than normal blood sugars also get "diabetic" neuropathy. It may be a major cause of the impotence so common among men in their 40s and older.

The pain of neuropathy usually starts out in your feet. It can feel like tingling or burning, though some people describe it as feeling like there is something stuck between their toes when there really isn't anything there.

Diabetic neuropathy differs from the nerve pain that can be caused by disc problems in the back in that it usually is symmetrical—i.e. it occurs in both feet. Less commonly, diabetic neuropathy can cause problems in the hands and arms.

Nerves affected by neuropathy eventually become numb. When you are examined after your diabetes diagnosis, your doctor should test your feet with a tuning fork or a thin filament that looks like fishing line to see if you have dead nerves in your feet that you may not have noticed. Many people with diabetes do. It is an important finding which tells the doctor that you are at risk for serious infections.

Neuropathy Affects More than Just Your Feet

While the nerves of your feet are the ones you are most likely to notice, the presence of neuropathy in your feet suggests that other nerves in your body are also under attack including the nerves of the autonomic system which control functions like blood pressure, heartbeat, sexual response, and the movement of food through your digestive system.

The more years you spend with high blood sugars, the more likely you are to develop sexual dysfunction. Neuropathy also leads to gastroparesis, the condition where food stays in your stomach for many hours because the nerves controlling the stomach values don't work properly.

Another nerve that gets damaged by high blood sugars is the vagus nerve, a vital nerve that connects your brain to the rest of your body. The vagus nerve has been found to play a major role in the regulation of the immune system. Neuropathic changes in the vagus nerve may have something to do with why people with diabetes have trouble fighting infections, since a weakened vagus nerve may not signal the immune system that your body is under attack.

The vagus nerve also regulates heartbeat. It is possible that damaged vagus nerves may have something to do with the high incidence of fatal heart attack in people with diabetes. Abnormal heartbeats may contribute to sudden cardiac death.

Neuropathy is painful, which is bad enough, but if it is allowed to progress, eventually it can lead to amputation. This may be partially because the death of nerves keeps the immune system from responding to infections and partially because what kills your nerves is the failure of the tiny blood vessels that supply them with nutrients. When your blood sugar is high for a long time, glucose clogs these tiny vessels and compromises blood flow. Nerves die from lack of nutrients and oxygen, germ fighting cells can't reach the infected tissue, and if the blood vessels in your limbs get clogged badly enough, you may develop gangrene.

So what has science found about the blood sugar level at which neuropathy starts to develop?

A lot. Several studies run by neurologists at different clinics discovered that the incidence of neuropathy starts to rise significantly in people whose blood sugar two hours after a oral glucose tolerance test is 140 mg/dl or over—i.e. people with prediabetes.

Neurologists at The University of Utah found that patients who were not known to be diabetic but who registered 140/mg or higher on the two hour sample taken during a glucose tolerance test, were much more likely to have the diabetic form of neuropathy than those who had lower blood sugars. Even more telling, the researchers found that *the length of time* a patient had experienced this nerve pain correlated with how high their blood sugar had risen *over* 140 mg/dl on the two hour glucose tolerance test.

What was also interesting about this study was that it found *no* correlation between the incidence of neuropathy and the two blood sugar tests most doctors who treat diabetes rely on to evaluate patient health. *Neuropathy did not correlate to any particular **fasting blood sugar level**, nor did it correlate to any particular **A1c value**.* But in people whose blood sugars were higher than 140 mg/dl two hours after they drank 75 grams of glucose there was a sudden significant increase in the incidence of diabetic neuropathy.

A second study performed by neurologists at Johns Hopkins confirmed these findings. Fifty-six percent of their patients who had neuropathy of unknown origin were found to have abnormal results on their oral glucose tolerance tests. The neurologist investigated the nerve damage further and learned that patients whose OGTT results fell in the prediabetic range had suffered damage to their *small* nerve fibers. The fully diabetic subjects whose OGTT results were over 200 mg/dl had more damage to their *large* nerve fibers. Yet another study, conducted at the Mayo Clinic in Scottsdale, AZ and published in August 2006 confirmed these results.

Anecdotally, many people who post about their experiences with diabetes on the Web have reported that they can make the pain in their feet go away by keeping their blood sugars under 140 mg/dl at all times, though if they let their blood sugar rise, the pain will come back. Some of those who control their blood sugar this way also find Alpha Lipoic Acid and Benfotiamine helpful for healing their nerves. We will discuss both in Chapter Ten.

Blood Sugar Level and Serious Illness

High blood sugars make you more prone to infection. So it is worth noting that a study found that when doctors kept the blood sugars of seriously ill hospitalized patients below 140 mg/dl at all times they improved their survival. A doctor working in an acute care setting was able to decrease the death rate of a group of critically ill patients by 29.3% simply by using insulin to keep their blood sugars below 140 mg/dl at all times.

This intervention also cut down the incidence of kidney failure and shortened the patients' stay in the ICU. In numbers this means that 45 people out of a group of 800 left the hospital alive who would have died had their doctor adhered to the ADA's far more lax definition of a "good" blood sugar target.

Blood Sugar Level and Beta Cell Dysfunction

Beta cells turn out to be very sensitive to slight rises in blood sugar. In fact, there's some evidence that beta cell dysfunction may begin when blood sugar spends more than a few hours at levels over 100 mg/dl.

A team of Italian researchers studying how the beta cells of normal people responded to rising glucose discovered that a small amount of beta cell dysfunction began to be detectable in people whose blood sugar rose only slightly over 100 mg/dl on a two hour glucose tolerance test.

Analyzing their data further, they found that with every small increase in the blood sugar concentration in the two hour glucose tolerance test there was a corresponding increase in how much beta cell failure was detectable. The higher a person's blood sugar rose within the "normal" range, the more beta cells were failing.

Another study found that beta cells start to die off in people whose *fasting* blood sugar is over 110 mg/dl. This finding is particularly striking since most doctors consider a fasting blood sugar of 110 mg/dl to be nothing to worry about. This may be related to the studies we looked at in Chapter Two that found that fasting blood sugar doesn't rise to 110 mg/dl until post-meal blood sugars have been high for several years. It is possible that it is not the mildly elevated fasting blood sugars that are killing beta cells, but the much higher post-meal blood sugars that are likely to be occurring when the fasting blood sugar has reached that level.

Which brings us back to the question of how high does blood sugar have to rise to kill a beta cell?

In mice, the answer seems to be *over 150 mg/dl*. Exposure to blood sugar concentrations that high turn out to kill transplanted beta cells that were previously healthy. Researchers working with mice receiving beta cell transplants showed that beta cell death was much lower in groups of mice receiving beta cell transplants whose blood sugar was kept under 150 mg/dl than it was in those who were allowed prolonged exposure to blood sugars higher than 150 mg/dl.[*]

But you're a man, not a mouse. It doesn't matter. A series of experiments done with cultured human cells found that prolonged exposure to high blood sugars kills human beta cells too. Furthermore, these experiments found that the higher the glucose level the beta cells were exposed to, the more dysfunctional they became. They also discovered that there was a time threshold beyond which the damage to beta cells caused by exposure to elevated blood sugars became irreversible.

The researchers took cells that had been damaged by exposure to high blood sugars and moved them to media that had a lower concentration of glucose. They found the cells could survive and recover after being moved to a growth medium containing a much lower concentration of glucose, but *only if the switch was made before a certain amount of time had passed*. Once the cells had been exposed to glucose for that fa-

---

[*] Normal and diabetic blood sugar levels in rodents are the same as they are in people, though there are important differences in how rodents metabolize glucose. Those differences explain why scientists have cured mice of diabetes hundreds of times without coming up with anything that works in humans.

tal time period, they could no longer be revived.

Though the study did not cite the specific blood sugar level at which damage occurred, I emailed the author of this study who wrote back, "I think the glucose toxic effects begin when blood glucose gets above 140 and probably earlier." However, he also explained that while studies with diabetic rats could better quantify the blood sugar levels at which this kind of irreversible damage occurs, these rats cost $200 apiece, and a lot of rats would be required, so they did not plan to do any further research on this topic.

Blood Sugar Level and Retinopathy

Retinopathy means "sick retina" and it is among the most terrifying of diabetic complications. What happens in retinopathy is that after extended exposure to high blood sugars the tiny blood vessels of the retina start to grow in a disordered manner. The retina is the part of the eye that contains the nerves that transmit light images to the brain.

These disordered diabetic blood vessels have weak walls, unlike healthy vessels, and eventually they burst, releasing blood into the eye. Left untreated, these overgrown vessels eventually destroy the optic nerve's ability to transmit images to the brain, resulting in permanent blindness.

Doctors currently treat retinopathy by using lasers to zap shut bleeding or swollen blood vessels in the eye. This helps retain vision, though it cannot restore nerves that have been destroyed by the blood vessel overgrowth.

It was long believed that diabetic retinopathy did not develop until blood sugar levels on the OGTT were well over 200 mg/dl. It was based on this belief that the American Diabetes Association's experts chose 200 mg/dl as the blood sugar to be used to diagnose diabetes, since they thought retinopathy only became a concern when blood sugars rose considerably higher than 200 mg/dl. Unfortunately, as is the case with so much of the data that the ADA's experts relied on to determine what blood sugar levels were safe, this turned out to be wrong.

A major study of a large population of people with prediabetes discovered retinopathic changes in the eyes of 1 out of every 12 people diagnosed with prediabetes. Even more significantly these people developed "diabetic" retinopathy even though they did *not* go on to develop blood sugars high enough to be diagnosed as diabetic.

The diagnostic criteria used in that study to define "prediabetic" was either a fasting plasma glucose that ranged between 100 and 125 mg/dl or a glucose tolerance test result that fell between 150 and 199 mg/dl.

Since, as we saw before, fasting blood sugars tend to rise only after post-meal blood sugars have been high for a while, this study's finding seems to suggest that exposure to post-meal blood sugars that remain over 150 mg/dl for two hours or longer is highly dangerous to your retina with or without a diabetes diagnosis, but even more so with a Type 2 Diabetes diagnosis.*

Do you see a pattern developing yet?

Blood Sugar Level and Cancer

Cancer cells have to eat too and glucose is their favorite food. Therefore it should come as no surprise that cancer rates rise significantly in people with "mildly" impaired blood sugars.

A Swedish study that followed 64,597 people for 10 years discovered that there was a very strong increase in the risk of cancer for those participants, no matter what their weight might be, who had fasting blood sugars over 110 mg/dl or who scored over 160 mg/dl two hours after a glucose tolerance test.

The risk continued to grow as participants moved into the diabetic category, but it did not increase by the same increment as it did when they moved from normal to what most doctors consider "mildly" impaired.

The cancers that responded the most strongly to exposure to higher blood sugars appear to be those of the pancreas, endometrium, urinary tract, and malignant melanoma.

Blood Sugar Levels and Heart Attack

It has long been known that people with diabetes have a much higher

---

* Many people with diabetes may mistake the blurry vision they experience when their blood sugar level fluctuate with retinopathy. In fact, blurry vision occurs because changes in the glucose concentration in the eye changes its refractive qualities. When you lower your blood sugar significantly, it is common to find you need to change your eyeglass prescription, especially if you are over 45. This does not mean you've damaged your vision. Retinopathy has no symptoms until you experience a bleed, at which point your visual field may fill up with black splotches. Make sure you get an eye exam as soon as you can after a diabetes diagnosis to determine if you have any signs of retinopathy. Laser treatments can prevent bleeds.

incidence of heart attack than does the rest of the population. But as was true with other "diabetic" complications, the damage starts at mildly elevated blood sugars. It turns out that heart attack risk more than doubles at blood sugar levels considered to be *prediabetic*.

Not only that, but if you are wondering about your own risk of heart attack, it turns out that your post-meal blood sugar levels predict the possibility of heart attack much more reliably than do your cholesterol test results.

Most people believe that high cholesterol predicts heart attack risk because this idea has been promoted very heavily in the marketing of the statin drugs that lower cholesterol. But it turns out that fully one half of all people who have heart attacks have normal cholesterol. Among those who have heart attacks who do have high cholesterol, analysis of the Framingham Heart Study data shows clearly that it isn't their LDL or total cholesterol levels that predict heart attack. It is their triglyceride levels and their ratio of total cholesterol to HDL.

What raises triglycerides? Dietary carbohydrate. What improves the ratio of total cholesterol to HDL? Lowering carbohydrates.

The oral diabetes medication Metformin will also significantly lower triglycerides.

A recent study found that triglycerides are stored in abnormal amounts in heart muscle very early in the progress of diabetes. This appears to occur at the blood sugar levels only slightly over normal — those defined as prediabetic. Statin drugs lower triglycerides only by a very small amount. The best way to lower triglycerides is to cut back on your carbohydrate intake.

A1c Accurately Predicts Heart Attack Risk

This astonishing finding was discovered a few years ago in a large-scale study called EPIC-Norfolk. What's particularly valuable about this study is that the researchers conducting it weren't looking for the causes of heart disease. They were studying cancer. Their finding that A1c predicted heart disease in people with supposedly normal blood sugar was a shocker.

Here's the summary from their published conclusions:

> In men and women, the relationship between hemoglobin A1c and cardiovascular disease (806 events) and between hemoglobin A1c and all-cause mortality (521 deaths) was continuous and significant throughout the whole distribution. The relationship was apparent in persons without known diabetes. Persons with hemoglobin A1c concentrations less than 5% had the lowest rates of cardiovascular disease and mortality.

In addition, the researchers concluded, "These relative risks were independent of age, body mass index, waist-to-hip ratio, systolic blood pressure, serum cholesterol concentration, cigarette smoking, and history of cardiovascular disease." In short, it wasn't their weight or their cholesterol that mattered. Blood sugar and blood sugar alone predicted whether or not a person was likely to have a heart attack.

Another study which drew similar conclusions discovered an even tighter correlation between A1c and heart disease risk that began as A1c rose above 4.6%, a level that is thought to correspond to an average blood sugar level near 86 mg/dl. This study found that the risk of heart attack doubled for every 1% rise in A1c. So a person with a 5.6% A1c had double the risk of someone with a 4.6% A1c. However, before you interpret this to mean that you are doomed, it is important to realize that "risk" is a statistical concept that exaggerates small differences.

It is illuminating to ignore "risk" and look at the actual *incidence* of the heart attacks reported in the EPIC-Norfolk study. As Table 3 shows, for every 100 men, there were 5 more cardiac "events," i.e. heart attacks, when the A1c of the group rose from 5% to 6%, but for women there was only an additional one and a half cardiac events per hundred when the group A1c rose by that amount. The published study notes that only slightly more than 20% of these cardiac events were fatal. This suggests to me that the 5% A1c range that most people with diabetes can attain without undue struggle greatly improves our chances of avoiding a heart attack.

Post-Meal Blood Sugars Predict Thickening in Carotid Artery Wall

More insight into why blood sugar might be so closely related to heart attack incidence was given by another study published by an Italian team in January of 2008. They reported that, in a group of people with diabetes who were measuring their blood sugar at home, the increase in the thickness of the carotid artery wall over five years correlated directly with how high their blood sugars rose after meals.

They found, too, that over the five year period 95% of the people with diabetes in their study experienced dramatic increases in the thickness of this vital artery. These people were being encouraged to eat a very high carbohydrate/low fat diet in the mistaken belief that it would prevent heart disease. As this study makes clear, it did not. The drugs these people were taking were unable to control their blood sugar peaks and the result was cardiovascular disaster.

A1c	<5.0%	5-5.4%	5.5-5.9%	6.0-6.4%	6.5-7.0%	>7.0%	Known Diabetes
Number of Men	1204	1606	1153	374	84	81	160
Coronary Events per 100 men	3.8	6.4	8.7	10.2	16.7	28.4	21.9
Number of Men's' Events	46	102	100	38	14	23	35
Number of Women	1562	1967	1378	439	73	68	83
Coronary Events/100 women	1.7	2.1	3.0	7.3	9.6	16.2	15.7
Number of Women's Events	26	41	41	32	7	11	13

Table 3. Actual Heart Attack Data from the EPIC-Norfolk Study

Post-Meal Blood Sugars Predict Heart Disease in "Normal" Women

Another intriguing study found a strong correlation between post-challenge blood sugar—i.e. post-meal blood sugar—and heart disease in a group of *normal* women. While there was no relationship between their *fasting* blood sugars and the rate at which they developed coronary artery disease over a period of about 3.5 years, there was a strong relationship between their scores on a *glucose tolerance test* and the degree to which they developed coronary artery disease.

Can Normalizing A1c Reduce Cardiac Risk?

Put on your seatbelts, we are about to enter a region of extreme turbulence. Two large studies published within weeks of each other in early 2008 came to dramatically different results on this question.

One, the ACCORD study, found that a population of people with diabetes and heart disease who followed an aggressive program of lowering blood sugar had slightly more heart attack deaths than a control group with laxer blood sugar control even though the group who followed the aggressive program attained an average A1c of 6.4%.

The second study, ADVANCE, which had enrolled twice as many subjects as ACCORD and lasted a longer time, found no increase in deaths in the group of participants treated more aggressively. They too attained an average A1c of 6.4%.

The reasons behind this discrepancy will only emerge when the data from these studies is published in peer-reviewed journals which may take years. We know from descriptions of the ACCORD study design published on the Web that the participants in the aggressive treatment arm of that study met regularly with dietitians who urged them to eat the high carbohydrate/low fat diet erroneously believed to prevent heart disease. They were given every possible drug to control blood sugar, including Avandia, Actos, and sulfonylurea drugs, all of which have been associated with an increased risk of heart attack or heart failure. They were also given Metformin and Byetta, a new drug whose long-term safety is unknown. On top of these, many were also put on the very high doses of insulin needed to counteract the very high carbohydrate diets they were prescribed.

In contrast, participants in the ADVANCE study were given only a single sulfonylurea drug and a single ACE inhibitor/diuretic drug to control blood pressure.

Though preliminary analyses of the ACCORD data supposedly did not point to any *one* drug as being at fault in the increased number of deaths, the use of so many drugs in a bewildering number of combinations and the interactions of all these drugs may have played a part in causing excess deaths. It is also possible that the use of the extremely large doses of insulin that were required to balance the very high carbohydrate consumption subjects in ACCORD were forced into may have promoted heart disease.

But whatever explanation eventually emerges for the differing results coming out of these studies, you are undoubtedly smart enough to have noticed that neither of these studies lowered blood sugar to anything approaching a normal level. The 6.4% A1c the aggressive control groups attained correlates roughly to an average blood sugar of 151 mg/dl. Since this is an *average* blood sugar, it is likely that participants were spending significant amounts of time above that ticipants were spending significant amounts of time above that level every time they ate. And as you can see from the chart summarizing the EPIC-Norfolk data, 6.4% is very close to the 6.5% level at which the incidence of heart attack took a huge upward leap.

There have been no large studies to investigate the effect on cardiac health of lowering the A1c below the much safer 5.5% level. Even more significantly, there are no large studies about what happens when you lower A1c by lowering carbohydrate intake rather than raising drug intake and resorting to huge doses of insulin.

Studies analyzing the low carbohydrate diet's efficacy for weight loss have found no increase in heart disease in low carbohydrate dieters who stayed with the diet for a two year period. But for now, there are no studies that can definitively answer whether lowering A1c to a truly normal level will give people a normal risk of heart disease, though the huge ADVANCE study shows that lowering the A1c level in and of itself should not be harmful.

And the Winner Is . . .

The data we've reviewed so far seems to point to the range between 140 and 160 mg/dl as being where organ damage begins to occur, at least in people who are routinely spending a few hours each day with blood sugars in this range. So it seems safe to conclude that it is repeated exposure to blood sugars between 140 and 160 mg/dl that make it more likely you will develop **microvascular complications** — retinopathy, neuropathy and possibly kidney damage. The data connecting blood sugar levels and thickening of the carotid artery and the relationship between A1c and heart attack also suggest that heart attacks are caused by long-term exposure to blood sugars in the 140-160 mg/dl range.

This is probably why the American Association of Clinical Endocrinologists currently recommends that people with diabetes try to keep their blood sugars under 140 mg/dl as much as possible. Sadly, the American Diabetes Association still tells people with diabetes that a blood sugar level of 180 mg/dl two hours after eating is "tight control" and suggests that this level is all people with diabetes need strive for.

The data correlating A1c to heart attack risk suggests that the very safest A1c is 4.7%, which is thought to correlate to an average blood sugar of 90 mg/dl. Heart attack risk starts to rise when A1c reaches 5.7% which is believed to correspond to an average blood sugar of 126 mg/dl, though as we saw, the incidence at that level, though it is greater than it is at 4.7% is not devastating.

Clearly, the lower you can get your blood sugar to go, the better. Avoiding fructose—which is present in grain and sugar—may help too. Many of us who have kept our post-meal blood sugar spikes low have found that if we eat much fructose it raises our A1cs higher than our blood glucose testing would otherwise predict.*

Now that you've reviewed the data about how blood sugar levels correlate with diabetic complications, you have the tools you need to decide what blood sugar level you must achieve to prevent any further damage to your body.

If you have been running very high blood sugars for a while, lowering your blood sugar to a safe level may seem like a daunting task. Don't worry! All people with diabetes can do far more than most doctors realize to lower their blood sugars, and most can bring their blood sugars down into the safe range using the techniques we'll be discussing in Chapters Six through Nine.

---

* Those of us who frequently measure our blood sugars after meals often find that our A1cs are frustratingly higher than expected. This is so common that it is a continual topic of discussion online. My guess is that because the formulas used to equate A1c to average blood sugar were derived from a population whose average A1c was well above 7%, the formulas break down when applied to people whose blood sugars are near normal. This may be because the lower your blood sugar, the longer your red blood cells are likely to live. If you'll recall, the longer a red blood cell lives, the more glucose it accumulates, and hence the higher the A1c reading.

Chapter Five
Must You Deteriorate?

The Toxic Myth Your Doctor Believes In

When you start to use the strategies you'll read about in the next couple chapters, wonderful things happen to your blood sugar. You stop experiencing the blood sugar swings that were making you hungry or crazy, you lose a couple pounds without trying, and life is starting to look good. A month later, you realize that your blood sugar is finally low enough that if the research cited here is right, maybe you won't have to lose your feet like Grandma did or go blind like Uncle Willy. Then, just when everything is going so well, you make the terrible mistake of confiding your enthusiasm to your doctor—who tells you not to get your hopes up, because no matter what they do, everyone with diabetes always deteriorates.

Congratulations. You've just run into the second toxic myth that kills and maims people with diabetes.

This toxic myth is the single most dangerous idea that you are likely to encounter as you begin your struggle to live a healthy life with diabetes. It is the belief that science has proven, beyond a doubt, that no matter what you do, your Type 2 Diabetes will get worse.

Your doctor almost certainly believes this. Though he may give lip service to the idea that you can control your disease through diet, exercise, and drugs, what he really believes is that nothing you can do will make much difference in your long-term outcome. This is why your doctor doesn't urge you to lower your blood sugar to normal levels, but merely writes you prescriptions for drugs that, at best, do a mediocre job of controlling your blood sugar. After all, why should he urge you to struggle and deprive yourself when the truth is that no matter what you do, you're doomed?

Why do doctors believe this? There are several reasons. Some will tell you that they've seen it in their practices. They'll tell you that they've treated lots of patients with Type 2 Diabetes and that few, if any, of their patients can control their diabetes with diet. They'll add that though they have counseled their patients to lose weight, their patients don't, and even those who have good control end up with complications.

If you challenge the doctor further, he's likely to tell you that it isn't just his patients, the research shows *everyone* with diabetes deteriorates regardless of how good their control might be and to back this up he will cite the one big study that doctors always cite when the topic of good control for people with Type 2 Diabetes comes up, the UKPDS.

Did the UKPDS Prove People with Good Control Still Deteriorate?

The **UKPDS** (United Kingdom Prospective Diabetes Study) was the largest, most exhaustive research study ever run to investigate what happens when people with Type 2 Diabetes improve their blood sugar control. It was an attempt to duplicate another landmark study, the **DCCT** (Diabetes Control and Complications Trial), which was a study of people with autoimmune *Type 1 Diabetes* which found that people with Type 1 Diabetes who maintained tight blood sugar control got far fewer diabetic complications than those with higher A1cs. Unfortunately, when it was complete, the UKPDS appeared to prove that tight control had far fewer benefits for people with *Type 2 Diabetes*.

Doctors will tell you that the UKPDS proved that the A1c test results of even the patients with good control gradually worsened every year. Not only that, but the UKPDS found that good control only made a small difference in the rate of complications, and that over the course of the study even the people with good control got lots of complications.

You can read a distinguished English diabetes expert telling exactly this to an audience of medical specialists in a lecture published by Medscape as part of an online course offered to doctors for Continuing Medical Education (CME) credit. In his presentation, Dr. Roy Taylor, a professor of medicine and metabolism at the University of Newcastle upon Tyne, points to a chart taken from UKPDS data titled "Newly Diagnosed Type 2 Diabetic Subjects Showing Progression of Retinopathy" and explains,

> These data are usually presented as showing a wonderful difference between the groups, [those controlling their blood sugar and those not] a 37% relative risk reduction. But take another look. This slope is unfortunate. This slope is almost equally unfortunate for the individuals concerned. Although intensive therapy in Type 2 Diabetes over 15 years makes a difference, it's not a staggering difference.

Later when he discusses the UKPDS findings about the progression of nerve damage he says "the abnormal nerve function continues to progress inexorably." When discussing early signs of kidney damage, he delivers the same message. "Intensive therapy [i.e. blood sugar control] does not seem to be able to stop this."

So it is no surprise that Doctor Taylor concludes that controlling blood sugar in Type 2 Diabetes may make a small difference,

> . . . but not such a huge difference that you would want to go out of your way as a patient to achieve it, perhaps, if you were shown this graph and told that over 15 years of intensive therapy you would be not much different compared with a "laissez faire" approach.

In short, this doctor is saying you might as well eat that donut, because no matter what you do, you're going to go blind anyway.

Abandon Hope All Ye Who Enter Here?

Is Dr. Taylor right? Logic suggests that if he is, you might as well enjoy that slice of cake while you can still see well enough to find your fork. If there is nothing you can do, it is rational behavior to shift your energy elsewhere and enjoy life—including the foods you love—while you can.

But in fact, this is *not* true. Doctor Taylor and his peers have missed one extremely important point in considering the UKPDS data.

Based on the findings of the research we reviewed in the previous chapters, *"Good Control" as defined in the UKPDS study was really mediocre control.*

Why? Because the definition of "good control" that was used in this study and, indeed, almost every study ever published, defined "good control" to mean that patients achieved A1cs of 7.0%.

When we apply the formula developed during the DCCT study that equates A1c with average blood sugar* and apply it to the 7.0% A1c that UKPDS defined as "good control," we quickly see why the UKPDS "good control" group is getting all those complications.

* The DCCT formula for equating average blood sugar level with A1c is:

Average Blood Glucose = (A1c * 35.6) - 77.3.

Another formula some doctors use is the Nathan Formula. It is:

Average Blood Glucose = (A1c * 33.3) - 86

The fact that these formulas come up with significantly different value and that doctors use both suggest that the A1c doesn't map down to average glucose as well as doctors would like to imagine it does.

That 7.0% A1c maps down to an average blood sugar of 172 mg/dl.

This blood sugar level is considerably higher than that 140 mg/dl level at which it appears that neuropathy and retinopathy begin and the level at which irreversible beta cell damage occurs.

But because the A1c reflects the *average* blood sugar but gives us no idea of the blood sugar *range*, the average blood sugar value the formula comes up with is deceptive. It does not distinguish between the person whose average blood sugar level of 172 mg/dl was achieved by maintaining their blood sugar at a steady 172 mg/dl throughout the day and the person who achieved that average with a blood sugar that surged up to 300 mg/dl, stayed there for three hours, and then plummeted to 70 mg/dl. Since the people in UKPDS were urged to eat a high carbohydrate/low fat diet and given large doses or insulin or drugs that stimulate the production of insulin, it is almost certain most of them were experiencing a pattern of high blood sugar peaks followed by low valleys.

So rather than proving that "good control" doesn't prevent complications, the UKPDS only proved that an average blood sugar of 172 mg/dl is toxic. Which you knew already.

Think of it this way: How would you feel if your doctor said that most patients who quit smoking develop lung cancer—after defining "quit smoking" as "smoked only 15 cigarettes a day?"

A Lesser-known Study Got Better Results than UKPDS

As we mentioned earlier, the A1c is only an average. It ignores the very important question of how high blood sugars are spiking after meals. So what happens if, instead of measuring only the A1c, you measure post-meal blood sugars and attempt to control how high they go?

A ground-breaking Japanese study of people with Type 2 Diabetes who were using insulin answered this question definitively. The researchers in this study, which was conducted in Kumamoto Japan, found that by lowering post-meal blood sugar targets, they were able to keep the A1cs of participants in their study stable over its entire six year course. Instead of the "inevitable decline" in A1c and blood sugar control that was seen in the UKPDS, the people with Type 2 Diabetes in the Kumamoto study saw no deterioration at all.

Not only that, but over the course of the study, the incidence of retinopathy, kidney damage, and nerve damage, was dramatically lower in the group that maintained tight control and that group as a whole saw slight improvements in their neuropathy by the end of the study rather than the deterioration seen in all other studies.

What makes this study so interesting is that the average A1c of the people in the Kumamoto "intensive intervention group" was *identical* to the average A1c of the people in the UKPDS study. What was different was that the blood sugar control strategy the Kumamoto study used focused *on keeping post-meal blood sugars lower.* So the Kumamoto study showed that *preventing high post-meal blood sugar spikes resulted in a much better health outcome, no matter what the resulting A1c.*

This is extremely good news for people who do not wish to succumb to inevitable decline. Especially since the patients in the Kumamoto study were aiming for a relatively high peak of 180 mg/dl after meals. That is low enough to improve insulin resistance and to stop the liver from dumping glucose inappropriately, but still much higher than the blood sugar level that should eliminate most diabetic complications.

A 2006 Study Proves Not All Type 2s Deteriorate and Some Even Improve

A long-term study of people with Type 2 Diabetes run at the Mayo Clinic measured the C-peptide levels of people with Type 2 Diabetes — C-peptide is an indicator of how much insulin they were still making — every two years over a period of twelve years. Here's what they found:

> Insulin secretion . . . declined with increasing duration of diabetes in approximately half of the patients *but either increased or remained essentially constant over time in the other half...* These data indicate that although a decrease in insulin secretion over time is characteristic of Type 2 Diabetes mellitus, it is not inevitable.

It is a shame they didn't tell us more about those people whose insulin production didn't decline or improved. Were they shooting for lower post-meal blood sugar targets? Eating a certain diet? Hitting the gym? Bowling? And did their insulin production increase because their insulin resistance was growing or because there was less stress on their beta cells? Without this information the study is not as informative as it might be. But like the Kumamoto study, it certainly answers the question," Do I have to deteriorate?" with a resounding, "No!"

All those Studies that Claim People with Diabetes Get . . .

Once you are diagnosed with diabetes, you will notice a steady stream of depressing stories in the media that report on studies that supposedly prove that people with diabetes are more likely to get everything from cancer to corns.

When you read these articles, remind yourself that almost every participant with diabetes in these studies had an A1c above 7.0% — it is usually *because* they have A1cs over 7.0% that they were considered diabetic by the scientists conducting the study — and that the conditions they came down with were not due to a specific disease, diabetes, but to their years of exposure to dangerously high blood sugars.

What Have Studies Learned About People Who Kept Their Post-Meal Blood Sugars Under 140 mg/dl?

So far, very little, because for decades doctors have been wedded to the idea that people with diabetes must eat a high carbohydrate/low fat diet to prevent heart disease. It is virtually impossible to attain post-meal blood sugars below 140 mg/dl eating a high carbohydrate diet.

Though research has discredited the ability of the low fat diet to prevent heart disease, all large scale studies of people with diabetes to date have encouraged the subjects to eat a very high carbohydrate diet and to limit their fat intake. So in all these studies, subjects ate meals that contained 75 to 100 grams of carbohydrate per meal and were then given drugs to counteract the blood sugar spikes caused by these high carbohydrate diets.

There is to date no large study of what happens when people with diabetes improve their post-meal blood sugars by using a significantly lowered carbohydrate intake with few or no drugs.

Since no large pharmaceutical company will make money selling low carbohydrate diets to people with diabetes, you probably won't see this kind of study anytime soon. Large studies are very expensive and the studies you see that involve many thousands of people are almost always funded in part by the big drug companies who hope that the study will prove that everyone with diabetes should be taking their drug.

The Choice is up to You

Since we can't point to rock solid research that proves that keeping your blood sugar under 140 mg/dl will completely eliminate complications, you might think you are taking a gamble by committing to that approach. But you are also taking a gamble if you don't. So the question you have to ask yourself is, "Which gamble has the highest cost if I'm wrong?"

If you pursue the regimen we recommend in the next chapters and achieve the blood sugar targets that we have suggested to you, and a decade hence some definitive study shows that even with excellent control and normal blood sugar levels patients still deteriorate, all that you'll have lost is a lot of carbohydrate-laden meals—and possibly some weight.

But if you settle for that 7.0% A1c your doctor recommends with its post-meal spikes over 200 mg/dl, and in ten years the studies show that keeping blood sugar under 140 mg/dl at all times *does* prevent most diabetic complications, you will have paid for your choice with bleeding retinas, failing kidneys, and gangrenous toes.

In addition, if lowering carbohydrates lets you lower your blood sugars to safe levels with few or no drugs, you are less likely to suffer from as the as-yet undiscovered dangerous long-term side effects of new diabetic drugs that won't be known for at least a decade.

So before you let your doctor give you a license to slack off, remember what is at stake: *it's not your doctor's retinas, kidneys, and toes that fail if your doctor is wrong.*

Chapter Six
How to Lower Blood Sugar

Now that you have a better understanding of what happened to you on your way to becoming diabetic, it's time to turn our attention to how you can get your blood sugar back to normal.

To do this is a multi-step process. The first step is to **change your diet** by cutting down the amount of carbohydrate you eat. This is the single most powerful tool you have with which to bring your blood sugar down to levels that are low enough to avoid any further damage to your body.

For many people, even those who were found to have extremely high blood sugars at diagnosis, cutting a lot of carbohydrates out of their diet is all they need to do to regain their health. We'll put a lot of effort into explaining how you can do this without making yourself crazy, because most of us have found that none of the other steps you can take to achieve normal blood sugars will work if you don't cut back on your carbohydrate intake.

If you cannot attain healthy blood sugars after you have eliminated the high carbohydrate meals that are so toxic to your beta cells, the next step is to work with your doctor to **see if any of the safer diabetes drugs might work for you**. In Chapter Eight we will explain to you everything you need to know to select such a drug from the list of those available.

If after adding one or two safe diabetes drugs to a diet that keeps carbohydrates under control you still can't get normal blood sugars, the final step, which *always* works, is to ask your doctor to help you craft **a modern insulin regimen.** This is an insulin regimen that restores your basal insulin release, and if you need it, your second-phase insulin release.* Don't shudder when you hear the word, "insulin." In Chapter Nine, we'll calm your fears about insulin and show you why

---

* Science has not yet come up with any insulin that will get to the bloodstream with the the speed of a natural first-phase insulin release. But if you go easy on the carbohydrates and eat only slow-digesting carbohydrates, you can get completely normal blood sugars using the second-phase insulin release you can restore with a well-crafted insulin regimen.

going on insulin early rather than late may be the smartest thing you will ever do for your health.

Harness the Power of an Effective Diabetes Diet

Diet is the most powerful tool available to you for restoring your body to normal health. But don't let the dreaded "D-word" fill you with foreboding or feelings of hopelessness. The diabetes diet we are going to be describing here has little in common with the restrictive ordeals you may have suffered through in the past in a vain attempt to lose weight.

The diabetes diet is not about calories. You are not going to have to starve yourself. You still get to eat dessert. The diabetes diet is not a low fat diet. It is not—despite what you have heard—a high protein diet. When you get your own personal diabetes diet working it will do two wonderful things for you: It will lower your blood sugar to a safe level and it will keep you from feeling hungry between meals.

The key words here are "your own personal diet." The diabetes diet that works for you is not necessarily the one that works for me. As we've stressed before, different things are broken in each of our metabolisms. So the goal of this chapter is not to tell you what to eat. Instead, what we are going to do is give you the tools and techniques you can use to design your own personal diabetes diet.

To do this, you're going to rely on three simple tools, your blood sugar meter, the log you will keep of your blood sugar test results, and a good reference that gives you nutritional information for the foods you eat. With these tools you'll be able to determine the exact diet that will make the best use of whatever beta cell function you have left. With these tools, you'll also be able to determine if diet is enough to restore your health or if you should investigate diabetes drugs. If you are taking a diabetes drug, you'll see how much impact it is having on your diabetes. If you exercise, you'll see how that exercise affects your blood sugar, too.

Using these tools will make you far less dependent on your doctor because you will know exactly how well your blood sugar is doing every day. When you visit your doctor you'll have clear blood sugar goals you want to attain and a good idea of how close you are to attaining them. You'll also be able to determine if your current doctor is willing and able to help you attain those goals or if it is time to look for a new doctor who will give you the support you need.

Your Power Tool: The Blood Sugar Meter

Your blood sugar meter is the single most powerful tool you have available to undo the damage caused by diabetes. In Chapter Four we reviewed the medical research that suggests that it is high post-meal blood sugars that damage your organs and, over time, lead to nerve death, amputation, blindness, and kidney failure. Your blood sugar meter can help you lower those post-meal blood sugars to the level where they stop damaging your body.

The way your blood sugar meter will help you do this is by showing you exactly what each meal you eat is doing to your blood sugar. It will help you see which foods are raising your blood sugar to danger-ous heights so you can eliminate them and replace them with other foods you enjoy that do not have that effect.

How to Choose a Blood Sugar Meter

People often start using a blood sugar meter because a pharmacy gave it away for free. But no matter what a blood sugar meter might cost, the significant expense associated with any meter is the cost of the **test strips** you must use each time you test your blood sugar. These strips are not reusable and they are extremely expensive.

Over the decade I've been using a meter, I've seen the cost of every other technology plummet to the point where I can buy a brand new computer that has a hundred times the power of my 1998 computer for one fifth of what I paid for that 1998 computer. But the price of test strips just keeps going up. Strips that were $.60 apiece in 1998 are now $1.03, and they aren't much more accurate now than they were ten years ago.

That means that unless you have premium health care coverage that gives you unlimited strips each month—which few of us do—you'll need a meter that uses strips you can afford.

In the United States you can buy a blood sugar meter without a pre-scription at any drug store. However, if your meter is going to be cov-ered by insurance, you may need a prescription from your doctor which specifies the exact brand. Many insurers will tell you which me-ter(s) they will cover at their lowest co-pay. Often it is the One Touch Ultra® or one of the Accu-Chek® meters. These are decent meters, and if your insurer helps pay for the strips, take them up on it. But their strips are the most expensive. So if you need more strips than your insurer will pay for over the course of one month, you'll want to buy a

MELANIE'S HAIR & NAI
1884 CURTNER AVE
SAN JOSE, CA 95124

TERMINAL I.D.:   SIG1
MERCHANT # :

01/29/10   2:04 PM

VISA
************3339
SWIPED

SALE
BATCH: 000232
INV:001014

AUTH: 04569B

BASE $116.00

TIP $_____

TOTAL $_____

TIP GUIDE
10% = $11.60 15% = $17.40 20% = $23.20

LAURIE E WARNER

CUSTOMER COPY

second, cheaper meter that uses cheaper strips.

The Relion® meter sold by Wal-Mart costs about $9 and the strips it uses cost less than half what the name brand strips cost. I have never received a report of these meters being any less accurate than the name brand meters which, as expensive as they are, have a spotty record for accuracy.

Another good choice is the TrueTrack® meter drug stores sell under their store brand name. Drug stores sometimes advertise promotions where they will give you a "free" drug store meter if you buy a box of 100 strips.

Some people report getting good results buying strips from sellers on eBay. I have done this myself. Just be sure that the expiration date on the strips hasn't passed. And don't ship strips when it is either very cold or very hot, as they may be damaged by exposure to temperature extremes.

Meters usually come with a lancet device, which is a spring-loaded object that looks like a pen. It's job is to shoot a thin metal spike into your finger just deep enough to draw blood. If the lancet device that comes with your meter seems painful, adjust the depth of the shot by twisting the barrel. If you still don't feel happy with it, you might find it worth investing in an Accu-Chek lancet device, as some of us find that lancet less painful than other brands.

Painless Blood Sugar Testing

If someone who doesn't themselves have diabetes taught you how to test your blood sugar, for example a nurse at a hospital or in your doctor's office, they may have taught you the wrong testing technique. This may be making testing unnecessary painful.

Here are some tips about how to test painlessly drawn from the experiences of dozens of people who have posted about blood sugar testing on the Web over the past decade.

Where to Test

The least painful spot to do a blood sugar test is on the side of your finger. Do not test on the pad of the finger. That hurts!

Many of us find that our pinkies have the best blood flow. I only use my pinky and ring fingers on both hands for testing.

Dr. Bernstein, the distinguished diabetes doctor and author who has had diabetes himself since 1946, recommends using the back of the finger, below the base of the nail. For me, that location hurts, so I don't use it.

Be sure to adjust the depth of your lancet to the shallowest depth before you test. That is usually "1" on most lancets. If that is too shallow to draw blood, adjust it up one notch and try again. As you get calluses on your fingers from testing, you may need to adjust the depth again. However, once you develop calluses your tests should become more painless.

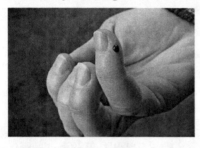

Figure 4. The least painful place to test

What About Testing on Your Arm?

Though many meters now offer the option of testing on your arm and promote this as if it were a benefit, many of us find that testing on our arms is more painful than using the sides of the fingers. And there is another more important problem: When you test your arm rather than your finger tip, the reading you get will lag about 15 minutes behind the reading you would have gotten using your finger tip. This is because the skin in your arm contains more interstitial fluid than your finger tips. It also means arm testing is worthless for detecting hypos.

Alcohol Toughens Skin

There is no need to dab your skin with alcohol before testing. Dr. Bernstein reports that neither he nor any of his patients has ever developed an infection after testing without alcohol. I have never used alcohol in nine and a half years and have never developed an infection from a blood test either.

The use of alcohol over time will dry out and toughen your skin, making it harder to draw blood. If your hand is dirty, wash it. If you see an unexpectedly high reading, you should also wash your hand and try again. A tiny bit of glucose or sugary food on your finger can cause dramatically high readings.

You Can Reuse Your Lancets

If you are the only person using your lancet device there is no need to use a fresh lancet for each test. I change mine once every few months.

Some people report changing theirs even less frequently. Many of us find used lancets are more comfortable to use than new ones.

Never Share a Lancet!

If someone else is going to share your lancing device—for example a relative interested in knowing whether their blood sugar is high after a meal—you must give them a fresh lancet and dispose of it immediately after they use it to avoid transmitting any blood borne diseases—including ones neither of you may be aware of. Never violate this policy!

Disposal of Test Strips

Blood products are considered medical waste. If you don't have access to a red bio-waste container, make one out of an old detergent bottle. When it is filled, tape the top closed and mark the container "Caution: Medical Waste." Then dispose of it according to your local trash ordinances. You can also buy inexpensive medical waste disposal units at most local pharmacies.

Meter Accuracy

There is a lot of misinformation floating around the Web about meter accuracy. You will often hear that meters may be off by as much as 20%. This is not actually true. While the standards that meter companies are required to meet *do* allow them to be off by 20%, in practice the meters sold now are usually much more accurate. Most of the time, when your blood sugar is near 100 mg/dl two meters of the same brand testing a drop of blood from the same puncture should give you a reading that is no more than 5 mg/dl different.

Meters from different companies may give readings that differ from each other by more than that. Anecdotally, people report that Accu-Cheks may give readings a bit higher than do One Touch Ultras.

Two readings taken on the same meter from two different punctures made as little as five minutes apart may also vary by a larger amount because the concentration of glucose in your blood can vary over that interval.

When your doctor schedules you for a fasting blood test, *bring your meter along and test right before the blood draw so you can compare your meter reading with the lab result.* That will give you a good idea of how accurate your meter actually is. Don't be concerned unless the difference between your meter and the lab is larger than 10%. At readings near 100 that would represent a difference of 10 mg/dl.

Any hint of inaccuracy is annoying in a device that uses disposables that cost what test strips cost. But for now you'll have to live with it. The meter's consistency with itself is the most important thing. If I know that my Ultra is 10 mg/dl lower than the lab result when my blood sugar is near 100 mg/dl, I can live with it. What I'm most interested in is how *high* my blood sugar rises after eating or how low it drops after taking insulin or another medication. The meter should portray that accurately.

If you get a meter that does not seem to be giving consistent results—and I have had one of those—contact the company and complain. They may replace it. Or take advantage of one of the free deals available at the drug store from time to time to get a new one. If your second meter of that brand isn't consistent, change brands.

If you wonder what the best brand might be at any given time, check with people who frequent Web diabetes discussion areas like Tudiabetes.com. Over time brands come and go, so today's best meter may not be the one most recommended next year.

If your meter requires coding, make sure that you have set the meter code to match the strip code before you test. This can make a big difference in accuracy.

Set a Healthy Blood Sugar Goal

The key to recovering your health is to select a set of healthy blood sugar targets and employ all the tools at your disposal to attain them. In Table 2 below you'll see four different blood sugar targets listed. In Chapter Four you read the scientific evidence that hints at what blood sugar levels damage your organs. Now it's time to commit to lowering your blood sugar below the level where that damage is likely to occur.

The targets given in Table 2 include post-meal blood sugar targets, A1c targets, and fasting blood sugar targets. Most of us find that if we lower our post-meal blood sugars enough to attain the post-meal targets, we will usually get an A1c in the recommended range. Lowering your post-meal blood sugars should also lower your fasting blood sugar. But fasting blood sugar is often the very hardest measurement to bring down to a normal level.

	CGMS Normal	5% Club	AACE	ADA
1 Hr after meal	120 mg/dl	Under 140 mg/dl	Not Given	Not Given
2 Hrs after Meal	85 mg/dl	Under 120 mg/dl	Under 140 mg/dl	Under 180 mg/dl
A1c Result	4.3% - 5.4%	5.0 - 5.9%	6.5%	7.0%
Fasting Blood Sugar	85 mg/dl	Under 110 mg/dl	Under 110 mg/dl	Under 130 mg/dl

Table 2. A Selection of Post-Meal Blood Sugar Targets

The most rigorous blood sugar targets are the True Normal targets derived from Dr. Christiansen's study described on Page 14 that used a continuous glucose monitor to examine the blood sugars of truly normal people. That target matches pretty closely the targets suggested by Dr. Richard K. Bernstein, who was the first to insist that people with diabetes could and should achieve truly normal blood sugars. These are the most rigorous blood sugar targets, but achieving them should eliminate any health problems caused by elevated blood sugars.

The next most rigorous set of blood sugar targets are those used by the people in the online diabetes community who call themselves "The 5% Club" because they strive to keep their A1cs in the 5% range. These are the blood sugar targets I shoot for myself. These targets are well below the levels associated with most diabetic complications. While they may be less than perfect, they are easily attainable even for a person like myself whose diabetes is caused largely by dysfunctional beta cells. And I can hit these targets without living a life of stringent self-denial. If you shoot for The 5% Club blood sugar targets you are very likely to end up with an A1c in the 5% range. I have.

The next set of targets, which are even laxer, are those suggested by the American Association of Clinical Endocrinologists (AACE). If you use the AACE targets you should end up with an A1c near that organization's recommended A1c of 6.5%. These targets come in barely under the levels that the research suggests damage organs.

The last blood sugar targets listed are the ones recommended the American Diabetes Association. Using them may result in your achieving an A1c in the 7% range that the ADA considers good enough for people with diabetes. People with A1cs of 7% still develop a lot of neuropathy, retinopathy, and other diabetic complications.

People often ask me what post-meal blood sugar goal they should shoot for. But let's get this straight. Your blood sugar goals are your blood sugar goals, not mine. So it is up to you to decide what blood sugar levels are acceptable. You're the person who has to do the work to reach those goals. You're the person who is going to suffer if they are wrong, or who may blow off the whole program if they are too stringent. I urge you to review the data you will read in Chapter Four very carefully before making your final decision about which blood sugar targets to shoot for.

Crafting Your Own Diabetes Diet

The first step to crafting your own individualized diabetes diet is to learn how high your blood sugar is rising after each meal when you are eating your usual diet. To start out, you won't make any changes to what you eat at all. All you will do is test after several of your usual meals so that you can observe how the foods you are currently eating affect your blood sugar. Here's what to do:

❖ **Measure your blood sugar before your meal.** Write down your pre-meal blood sugar reading on a blood sugar log of some type. You may want to use the little book that comes with your meter or you may just keep track on a piece of paper. If you enjoy technology, you can create a spreadsheet or you can find sites on the Web that will help you keep track your blood sugar and graph it. Note the date and time along with your blood sugar reading.

❖ **Eat a meal made up of foods you routinely eat.** Note the time on the clock when you finished eating your meal. Be sure to write a note about what you ate in this meal. If there isn't enough room to describe the food in your meal in your log, write it down in a notebook with a note about the time when you ate it or write yourself an email noting what you ate. It is very important to be able to link the blood sugar you measure after a meal with information about what food was in that meal.

❖ **Test your blood sugar one hour after you finished your meal.** Write your blood sugar test result in your blood sugar log along with the time that you tested.

❖ **Test your blood sugar two hours after you finish your meal.** Again, write down the results in your log along with the time.

Test a typical lunch and a typical dinner. Then test a breakfast. Do this until you have accumulated test results for six or seven meals you frequently eat.

After you test a few meals, you should start to notice when your highest blood sugar occurs after a meal. For many of us it is about an hour after eating. If your access to strips is limited, you may decide only to test at that time. Or you may alternate between testing at one and two hours.

What Raised Your Blood Sugar?

Take a look at your test results and pick out all the meals that raised your blood sugar over your chosen blood sugar targets. If that's all of them, don't worry. Most people with diabetes will see blood sugar values that are going into the 200s or higher after just about every meal. That's what got them diagnosed as diabetic!*

Now it's time to face an important fact. *It is the carbohydrates you eat that raise your blood sugar after meals.* Sugars and starches. Nothing else.

The fats you eat do not raise your blood sugar at all. Technically speaking, protein *can* raise your blood sugar because your liver is able to convert about 58% of the protein you eat into carbohydrate. But since it takes up to seven hours to digest dietary protein and turn it into glucose, the only people who see a rise in blood sugar after eating protein are those whose diabetes is so severe that they have no beta cell function left at all. So it is unlikely that eating protein will cause an observable rise in your blood sugar.

But every gram of carbohydrate you eat, whether it comes from

---

* If your blood sugars are normal after meals, and you are only diabetic in the fasting state, this is important information. It is still worth testing to see what happens to your fasting blood sugar when you lower your carbohydrate intake for a week or two. But if that doesn't make a dramatic change in your fasting blood sugar, you will probably have to turn to medications to lower it.

sugar, bread, potato, pasta, fruit, "low glycemic foods," or what the food industry likes to call "healthy whole grains," *will* turn into glucose once it is digested. And as soon as that glucose enters your bloodstream it will raise your blood sugar. When it does, you experience what we call a **blood sugar spike**.

Use your nutritional reference to figure out how many grams of carbohydrate there were in the three meals that raised your blood sugar the highest. Now it is time to see how much you can lower your postmeal blood sugar spikes by lowering the amount of carbohydrate in each of those meals.

There are two ways of doing this. You can plunge right in or edge in gradually. We'll explain how to do both.

Special Considerations When You Are on Insulin or a Drug That Increases Insulin Production

Plunging right in can lower blood sugars dramatically. If you are currently injecting insulin or if you are taking an oral drug that forces your beta cells to produce insulin, you will need to proceed cautiously and talk to your doctor about how you should reduce the doses of these drugs as your diet lowers your blood sugar. Otherwise you may risk dangerous low blood sugars.

So if you are using insulin or a drug that causes your beta cells to produce insulin, use the second technique described here, "Inching in slowly." With that approach, you can lower your medication gradually.

The oral drugs that increase insulin production are the drugs in the sulfonylurea family. They include Glipizide (brand name: Glucotrol), Glyburide (Micronase, DiaBeta, Glynase), and Glimeprimide (Amaryl). Two other drugs that behave in a similar manner are Starlix and Prandin. The other commonly prescribed diabetes drugs, Metformin, Avandia, Actos, Januvia, and Byetta should not cause hypos, so if you are taking one of these, you can adopt either approach.

Learn How Much Carbohydrate is in Your Food

The key to improving your diet is learning how much carbohydrate there is in the foods you usually eat. So pick up a book of food counts at your local library or bookstore. Start browsing through it. Look up the foods you usually eat and see how many grams of carbohydrate there is in a single portion. The carbohydrate content of foods is always given in grams. There are 28.3 grams in an ounce.

A books of nutritional information, like one of those written by Corinne T. Netzer, is a good place to start learning about the carbohydrate content of your foods because you can leaf through a book and scan the nutritional information it contains quickly. That way you can discover foods with a low carbohydrate content that you might not have thought of looking up.

When you want to look up a specific food or calculate the nutrients in a complex meal, nutritional software can be very helpful. Download useful shareware software from **lifeform.com** or **calorieking.com**.
If you like it, you can register it for a modest sum. I find it invaluable. Other people recommend the nutritional software found on the Web at: **fitday.com**

These software tools will compute the amount of carbohydrates and other nutrients in your meal for you, as long as you know the portion size. You can also look up the nutritional content of foods on the USDA Web site at: **nal.usda.gov/fnic/foodcomp/search/**

Portion Size Matters

When you look up the carbohydrate count of a food, you must pay attention to the portion size to which that count applies. If your favorite muffin weighs six ounces, don't kid yourself that it has only 22 grams of carbohydrate. Yes, that may be the carbohydrate count you see listed in your nutritional guide for the entry, "blueberry muffin," but the portion size for muffins given in nutritional guides is almost always two ounces. Those huge muffins you find at your local coffee shop may weight up to eight ounces each and contain between 60 and 100 grams of carbohydrate each.

You can also learn a lot about the carbohydrates in your food by reading the nutritional panels you'll find on boxed and canned foods. Again, note the portion size. Have you ever gotten 2.5 servings out of a can of Campbell's Soup? Me neither, but that's the portion size listed on the can.

An electronic food scale can be very helpful. Buy one and weigh the foods you eat at home for a few weeks until you get the hang of estimating portion size. Where the nutritional label printed on a processed food gives you both a weight and a measurement like "one half cup," the weight is always more accurate than the volume measurement. You can get a good food scale at a gourmet kitchen shop. Though they are expensive, a food scale may be the best nutritional investment you'll ever make. When you weigh a serving of ice cream on a food scale, you'll quickly see that the "one serving" listed on the package turns out to be only a few teaspoons' worth. That bowl you've been considering as one portion of ice cream weighs in at four servings, which turns out to be 72 grams of carbohydrate and 600 calories. That may explain its damaging effect on both your blood sugar and your waistline.

This may sound like a lot of work, and when you first start out, it is. But after a few weeks you'll have memorized the gram counts and the portion sizes for most of the foods you usually eat. Soon you won't have to test every time you eat a favorite meal, because you will know beforehand exactly what it will do to your blood sugar. You'll also be able to estimate the impact of a new food on your blood sugar just by looking it up, because you will know by then how high your blood sugar rises after you eat a certain number of grams of carbohydrate.

Craft Your Diet by Plunging Right In

Now that your tools are ready for use, it's time to get to work on your blood sugars. The fastest way to do this is to remove all the carbohydrates from one of the meals you've just tested and see what that meal does to your blood sugar when you eat it without any carbohydrates.

If you ate a burger, fries, and salad, for example, try eating only the burger without the bun and the salad. Instead of a sugary salad dressing such as a raspberry vinaigrette, try oil and vinegar, Italian, blue cheese dressing, or maybe ranch or parmesan peppercorn. All these are low in carbohydrate.

If a meal contains almost nothing but carbohydrates, for example, a breakfast of cereal, milk, and toast, try eating a different meal that contains almost no carbohydrates, such as eggs and ham without toast. Don't worry about fat content. If you are not eating carbohydrate, fats won't hurt you and they won't cause weight gain.

Test your no-carbohydrate or almost-no-carbohydrate meal one hour after eating and again two hours after eating, to see how the blood sugar spike that follows your reduced carbohydrate meal compares with the one you saw after eating the high carbohydrate version.

If you are like most people, you'll see a dramatic difference. Now remove the carbohydrates from the rest of the meals you tested earlier that raised your blood sugar very high. Keep doing this for at least two weeks. It takes a while for high blood sugars to drift down, but by the end of two weeks you should be seeing blood sugars much better than those you started out with.

As you lower the carbohydrate content of your meals, start adding to your daily diet several portions of low carbohydrate vegetables such as green beans, artichokes, asparagus, lettuce, spinach, brussels sprouts, broccoli, and cauliflower. Keep testing. These vegetables should not raise your blood sugars.* Add low carbohydrate berries too. Raspberries, strawberries, and blueberries eaten in moderation should not raise your blood sugar.

Learn More About Successful Low Carbohydrate Dieting

The lowered blood sugars you see after cutting out the carbohydrates may be enough to motivate you to go on a very low carbohydrate diet for a while, which is an excellent way to drop your blood sugars to normal levels very quickly. A very low carbohydrate diet rich in vegetables and berries is a safe and very effective way to normalize your blood sugars.

Unlike most diabetes drugs, the low carbohydrate diet has never been proven to cause serious side effects. Besides lowering your blood sugar dramatically, a few months on a very low carbohydrate diet, should give you improved blood pressure, cholesterol, and triglycerides.† Though some studies of people with *normal* metabolisms have found no weight loss difference between low carbohydrate diets and other kinds of diets, other research has shown that the low carbohydrate diet is more effective at producing weight loss in people who are insulin resistant.

The diets described in the books *Protein Power* and *Dr. Bernstein's Diabetes Solution* are both safe and effective ways to normalize your blood sugars very quickly. Either diet will probably also take weight

* If your blood sugars rise significantly after eating only the carbohydrates found in truly low carbohydrate vegetables, you may need to see an endocrinologist or a doctor skilled in prescribing insulin, as that would suggest you are making almost no insulin at all.

† Some people will see a brief rise in cholesterol levels when they start a low carbohydrate diet, usually because they will also start losing weight. Cholesterol rises early in most weight loss diets. Don't worry about your cholesterol levels until you have been eating that way for six months or so. The theory that eating fat causes heart disease has been discredited. Eating carbohydrates turns out to be what worsens the important cholesterol values, not eating fat. Over time, lowering your carbohydrate intake will drop your triglyceride count dramatically.

off you too, especially if your only previous experience with dieting has been low fat dieting. Reading a variety of books about low carbohydrate dieting can give you more insight into strategies for making your diet work.

Hunger

The first two or three days after you've cut carbohydrates out of your meals, you are likely to be very hungry. This is because your blood sugar will be dropping rapidly and your body is not used to that happening.

But if you can get through those two or three days your blood sugars will stabilize at a lower level and the hunger should dissappear. What you should then experience is a new and delightful feeling of *freedom from hunger*. It is surprising how few days it takes for this to happen. So if you are hungry after eating your first few very low carbohydrate meals, tell yourself that the hunger is temporary, commit to sticking with the program for three days, and see how you feel when those three days are over.

If you want to snack, eat low carbohydrate snacks like cheese, sunflower seeds, meat, or one of the low carbohydrate treats you'll find on Page 178.

Raising Your Carbohydrate Intake

Some people are extremely happy with how they feel while eating a very low carbohydrate diet. Others are not. It will take at least two weeks until you can evaluate the effect of a very low carbohydate diet on your own, unique metabolism.

If you decide after a few weeks of eating a very low carbohydrate diet that this is not how you want to keep on eating, your next step should be to start testing your meals to see how much carbohydrate you can add back before your blood sugar rises back into the danger zone.

Try adding five more grams of carbohydrate to one of your very low carbohydrate lunches or dinners.* Test that meal one and two hours after you eat it and see what happens. If you are still well below your chosen blood sugar target, add an additional five grams of carbohydrate to your next meal. Continue adding carbohydrate until you dis-

---

* Most people, including those with completely normal blood sugars, are more insulin resistant at breakfast than at any other time of the day. So expect higher readings then.

cover the amount of carbohydrate that pushes your blood sugar over your chosen blood sugar target.

If it turns out that intake level is very low, don't panic. A well-chosen diabetes medication may allow you to raise your carbohydrate intake to where it is tolerable.

Craft Your Diet by Inching In Slowly

The other approach many people find helpful for getting back their blood sugar control is the inverse of the technique we just described. Here you take a meal that raised your blood sugar too high for safety and start whittling away at the carbohydrates it contains a little bit at a time.

So if your original meal was a hamburger, fries, and a salad, you would try the same meal without a bun. Test your blood sugar one and two hours after you finish eating, log your results, and see how much of an improvement you made by losing the bun. If you are seeing blood sugars higher than your target, try cutting out half the fries. Test again. If you are still over your target, eliminate the rest of the fries, or swap your sugary salad dressing and croutons for a low carbohydrate dressing.

If your breakfast of cereal and milk isn't working, try replacing the cereal with steel cut oatmeal. If that doesn't help, try a low carbohydrate flax cereal. Still too high? Try using a low carbohydrate milk product like that sold under the name "Calorie Countdown" instead of low fat or regular milk. If you still can't get a good reading, you'll have to take cereal off the menu. Try eating a low carbohydrate breakfast like eggs and meat instead.

With this technique you can eat whatever you want—as long as you can reach the blood sugar targets you have set for yourself.

Undoing the Damage Done by High Blood Sugars

As you read earlier, if you have been running very high blood sugars for many weeks or months, long-term exposure to these high blood sugars will have greatly increased the strength of your insulin resistance. This makes whatever insulin your beta cells can make much less effective.

If your liver has become insulin resistant too, which often happens, it may be dumping extra glucose into your bloodstream at meal times, because it can't detect the insulin signal that should be telling it that blood sugars are high enough.

The great news for you is that by lowering your carbohydrate intake, you can reduce your insulin resistance. If you achieve any of the blood sugar targets you saw in Table 2, after a few days your insulin resistance will start to decrease. Then whatever insulin you are still making will work more effectively, so that even without growing a single new beta cell, you will get a lower rise in blood sugar from each gram of carbohydrate you eat.

Even better, as your insulin resistance decreases, your liver may also become less insulin resistant and stop dumping loads of unneeded glucose into your bloodstream. This, too, will bring your blood sugars down dramatically.

What Can You Achieve?

Surprisingly, how high your blood sugar is when you start this program does not predict how fast your blood sugars will drop or how many grams of carbohydrate you will end up being able to eat safely. I have seen people with extremely high blood sugars eat twice the amount of carbohydrate I eat and end up with blood sugars better than any I have ever been able to attain.

Your size and gender have a lot to do with it. The larger you are, the more carbohydrate your body can handle. Men typically can handle a bit more than women of the same size, possibly because they tend to have more muscle mass and muscle is what burns off the most glucose.

The other factor that determines how far and fast you can progress is the degree to which your diabetes is caused by irreversible beta cell dysfunction. If you have enough functional beta cells left, lowering insulin resistance will make a huge difference in your blood sugars. If, like me, your beta cells don't secrete insulin properly, or if your beta cells are dead, the amount of carbohydrate you can cover with the insulin you still make will be very limited.

But there is really no way to know if your problem is insulin resistance, insulin insufficiency, or a mixture of the two until you start lowering your carbohydrate intake and see what happens. For many people, what happens is a very pleasant surprise. They achieve blood sugar numbers far better than what their doctor told them would be possible, and do it without any need for medication.

For them, lowering the carbohydrate intake is all that is needed to normalize blood sugar. For others it will be the first step, but other steps will have to follow. But it *is* the first step, so get yourself a meter and get testing!

False Hypos

As your blood sugar starts dropping towards the normal range, you may start experiencing low blood sugar symptoms. You may feel shaky or panicky a few hours after eating. At that point, you may fear you are heading for a dangerous low blood sugar attack and be tempted to eat some carbohydrates to raise your blood sugar back up.

Don't jump to the conclusion you are having a low blood sugar attack! Test your blood sugar. If it is over 70 mg/dl, reassure yourself that what you are experiencing is **normal blood sugar**. *If you are not injecting insulin or taking a sulfonylurea drug you do not have to worry about hypos!*

The word "hypo" is short for "hypoglycemia," which in turn is mangled medical-Greek for "low sugar." A true hypo is an emergency that occurs when too much insulin in your bloodstream causes your blood sugar drop so low that your brain cannot function.

But if you are not using insulin or insulin stimulating drugs, you are not at risk for dangerous hypos. Neither Metformin, Byetta, Januvia, Acarbose, Avandia nor Actos cause dangerous hypos. Nor are hypos a problem for most people who are controlling their blood sugar using diet alone.

What you are likely to encounter as you lower your blood sugar is a **false hypo**. The false hypo makes you feel as if you were having a severe attack of low blood sugar, but while it is uncomfortable, it is not a crisis. It is, in fact, a well-understood phenomenon that can happen if your fasting blood sugar has been elevated above truly normal levels for any period of time.

To understand the difference between a real hypo and a false hypo, you need to understand that a truly normal fasting blood sugar may range from 70 mg/dl up to the low 90s. That blood sugars as low as 70 mg/dl are safe is shown by the fact that doctors recommend that pregnant women keep their fasting blood sugars between 60 mg/dl and 90 mg/dl. So a blood sugar in the 60-70 mg/dl range is not a life-threatening emergency!

Hypos only become dangerous when blood sugar starts to drop into the 50s or lower. If your blood sugar drops into the 20s for any extended period of time you can become unconscious. This kind of hypo is a huge problem for people who inject too much insulin or take too much of an insulin-stimulating drug. But the only time a truly dangerous hypo will happen to a person who is not injecting insulin or taking an insulin-stimulating drug is if they have a rare endocrine disorder.

The reason you don't have to fear a hypo if you are not artificially raising your insulin level is that your body has an exquisitely sensitive feedback system whose job is to push your blood sugar back up as soon as it has dropped to more than 20 or 30 mg/dl below your usual fasting blood sugar level. When this happens, this system kicks in with dramatic effect.

It does this by secreting "counter-regulatory hormones" which are your old friends the "fight or flight" stress hormones. One good burst of counter-regulatory hormone and your blood sugar will surge back into the safe zone. Unfortunately, that burst of counter-regulatory hormone can also get your pulse pounding, your sweat glands pouring, and your body feeling as if you'd just narrowly escaped becoming a predator's lunch.

What makes the counter-regulatory response so hard to deal with for Type 2s—and what adds to the confusion about the danger of hypos—is that the body does not have a set, *absolute* threshold for responding to perceived hypos. It does not say to itself, "Uh-oh, blood sugar approaching 55, time to do Hypo Repair!"

Instead, it uses a *relative* threshold based on the fasting blood sugar level it is accustomed to. If you've been running a fasting blood sugar of 180 mg/dl for a while and then cut back on your carbohydrates for a few days, when your blood sugar drifts down to 120 mg/dl, your body may scream, "Blood sugar 60 mg/dl below normal! Hypo! Hypo!" even though your blood sugar is barely approaching a normal level.

When your heart is pounding, and you are feeling shaky and faint, it is very tough to do nothing, especially since your brain is likely to be sending out signals to the effect that all would be well if you'd just scarf down some nice, high carbohydrate food to "fix" the problem.

Don't!

Instead, when you feel hypo, grab your blood sugar meter and test. Unless your blood sugar is under 70 mg/dl don't do anything. It is not unusual to experience the symptoms of a false hypo, test, and discover that your blood sugar is actually *higher* than your usual fasting level.

The reason this happens is that, by the time you feel the impact of those stress hormones, they have already forced your liver to dump a load of glucose into your bloodstream to raise your blood sugar. This raises your blood sugar. Even worse, the stress hormones not only leave you feeling jangled, they may make you even more insulin resistant than usual for the next couple hours.

This false hypo response can be a major barrier on the road to achieving normal blood sugars. If you aren't prepared for it, you may end up sabotaging yourself by reacting to the symptoms of a false hypo by gobbling carbohydrates in the belief that you are fighting a life threatening hypo.

The best way to deal with this is to know that the body will reset its glucose "thermostat" over time. If you don't treat a false hypo as if it were an emergency, your body will eventually get used to a new, lower, fasting blood sugar. Then it will only give hypo signals when you are truly hypo—which if you are a Type 2 who is not using insulin or insulin-stimulating medications will never happen.

When the adjustment is complete, and your body gets used to living with normal blood sugars, you'll feel far better than you did in the past when your blood sugar was high. The only "problem" you may then encounter is that if you eat the way you used to, the very high blood sugar levels you used to feel comfortable at, now feel horribly toxic. This is actually good, because that unpleasant feeling when your blood sugar rises into the danger zone will motivate you to keep yourself from eating the foods that cause those damaging highs.*

---

* Online surveys have turned up the interesting finding that about half of all people with diabetes feel toxic when their blood sugars are high, but the other half can't feel high blood sugars.

Chapter Seven
Making Your Diet Work

Okay, you've been using your meter to check out your meals, and it's starting to hit you that yes, it is those carbohydrates that are raising your blood sugar. Even better, when you cut back on the carbohydrates your blood sugar starts to drop dramatically and you begin to experience blood sugars far better than any you have seen since your diagnosis. But if your previous experience with restricting carbohydrates was a weight loss diet which worked well for you until you crashed off it entirely and gained back all the weight you'd lost, you may be hesitant to embark on another course of dieting that requires that you commit to restricting your carbohydrate intake.

If so, join the crowd. Sticking to a stringent diet is always a challenge. Doing it when there is no end in sight, no weight loss goal to look forward to when you can hope you will be able to eat less stringently, is even harder. So unlike all the other authors who promote low carbohydrate diets, I am not going to tell you that you will feel so great on the diet that you will adhere to it for the rest of your life and never have any problems sticking to it.

Maybe you will. I know a few people who have. But after years of reading the messages posted daily on the low carbohydrate diet newsgroup and even more years reading the diabetes discussion forums, my guess is that like most people who adopt long-term low carbohydrate diets you *will* run into problems—the same problems that derail most people who adopt these diets. So what I'm going to tell you now is that you should *expect* these problems and build into your diet some strategies to solve them.

Weight Loss Diets Fail but Diabetes Diets Can't Afford To

Despite the rosy picture painted in all diet books, most people who adopt a low carbohydrate diet in order to lose weight fail. They start out with great enthusiasm and during the early period when they are losing weight they swear they will never again eat another French fry or piece of toast. Some stick to their diets for months or even years. But after denying themselves so many of the foods everyone else around them is eating, most eventually burn out and slink back to their old eating patterns, usually gaining back all the weight they lost and more.

This is not a surprise. People on *any* diet — including a low calorie or low fat diet — do the same thing. The body is very resistant to weight loss. Instincts buried deeply in our brains do everything they can to raise our weight back to where it used to be, no matter how unhealthy that weight might have been. But while a failed diet may be tolerable for those who are dieting to shed a few pounds before their class reunion, it spells disaster when we must change our diet to prevent amputation, blindness, kidney failure, and heart attack death.

Eating a low carbohydrate diet for diabetes means eating low carbohydrate for life — long after the thrill has worn off of eating all that yummy cheese and steak. Despite the hype in the diet books, it is not easy, simple, and fun. After many years of participation in low carbohydrate diet support groups on the Web, I have met only a handful of people who have been able to sustain a stringent ultra low carbohydrate lifestyle for more than five years.

But what I have observed over the same period of time is that there are a lot of people with diabetes who do the diet in a different way, and these people *have* been able to make a carbohydrate restricted diet work through years and even decades. They succeed because the approach they take is different in subtle ways from that of the weight loss dieter. Now let's look at how they do it.

The Tricks That Make a Life-Long Diabetes Diet Work

Focus on Your Blood Sugar Targets, Not Grams

When people think about adopting a lower carbohydrate diet, their first question is almost always, "How many grams of carbohydrates can I eat at each meal?" Most of the diet books will answer that question with a hard and fast number. Atkins, for example, tells you to start out with 20 grams a day. *Protein Power* starts you at 30 grams. Dr. Bernstein suggests that you eat 6 grams for breakfast and snacks and 12 grams at lunch and dinner.

Adopting these very low carbohydrate limits will control your blood sugar very nicely. But over time, many people find that sticking to a diet this low in carbohydrate becomes impossible. That's why the approach we sketched out in Chapter Six did not tell you how many grams to eat. Instead all you have to do is eat the number of grams of carbohydrate that lets you meet the blood sugar targets you have set for yourself.

This is what The 5% Club calls **eating to your meter**. What you're doing when you eat to your meter is creating what Australian newsgroup activist Alan S. calls *a low spike diet* rather than a low carbohydrate diet. Alan reports that he is able to keep his blood sugars under 140 mg/dl even when eating as many as 30 or 40 grams of carbohydrates at a meal. Other people with diabetes report that they must eat a lot fewer grams of carbohydrate than Alan eats to achieve safe post-meal blood sugar targets. But no matter how many grams they are eating, the result is the same: one hour post-meal blood sugars under 140 mg/dl.

The reason why Alan can eat almost three times as many grams of carbohydrates as I can is something that diet books rarely mention, though it is explained in detail in the book, *Dr. Bernstein's Diabetes Solution*. The explanation is that the amount of carbohydrate you can manage has a lot to do with your body size. The more you weigh, the less each gram of carbohydrate you eat will raise your blood sugar. The same two grams of carbohydrate that will raise the blood sugar of a person who weighs 280 lbs only 5 mg/dl will raise the blood sugar of a person who weighs 140 lbs a full 10 mg/dl—twice as high.

In addition, as we saw earlier, some of us are diabetic because of high insulin resistance, some because our beta cells have stopped secreting first or even second-phase insulin, and some because our beta cells have stopped secreting basal insulin. The nature and extent of the damage to our bodies will determine how much carbohydrate we can clear without spiking. The only way you will learn this is by testing the meals you eat with your meter and modifying those that raise your blood sugar over the blood sugar targets you have chosen.

Through testing after meals you'll learn how many grams of carbohydrate your own, unique, body can handle. And more importantly, you'll also be able to decide if your body can handle enough grams of carbohydrate that it will be possible to control your blood sugar through diet alone, or whether you will need to talk to your doctor about supplementing dietary control with drugs.

Eating Away from Home

The biggest challenge you'll encounter as you change your diet to lower your blood sugar will be eating away from home. You aren't going to be able to weigh restaurant foods nor can you look up the nutritional values of many restaurant offerings. That makes it a very good idea to avoid starchy or sugary restaurant foods or, if you do eat them, to eat only a small portion of what you are offered. Measure your blood sugar an hour or two hours after eating if you aren't sure about how a restaurant food will affect you. Then the next time you visit that restaurant you'll have a better idea of what to order.

Some Foods Give Misleading Test Results

Carbohydrates Eaten with a Lot of Fat will Digest Slowly

Foods with a lot of fat in them take longer to digest than those without a lot of fat. This is why pizza and ice cream often give deceptively good readings on your meter. If you test a meal and see a reading that is too good to be true, be sure you test at 3 or four hours after eating.

One thing to keep in mind is that eating a lot of fat is only healthy if you aren't eating a lot of carbohydrate and if you aren't producing, or injecting, a lot of insulin. Insulin turns excess carbohydrate into fat, so the more carbohydrates you eat, the less fat you should eat, no matter what your blood sugar is after the meal. It is also likely that the combination of a lot of carbohydrate and a lot of fat may have the evil impact on heart health previously attributed to fat alone.

The Truth About Pasta

Pasta was long recommended to people with diabetes as a food that would not raise blood sugar. This is why you will still see it starring in many cookbooks and magazines intended for people with diabetes.

Pasta usually doesn't raise blood sugar one hour after you eat and rarely after two. But if you test four or five hours after eating that pasta, you may get an unpleasant surprise. This is true even of the so-called "low carb" pastas. Pastas give you excellent readings at one and two hours because they are resistant to digestion, so they don't turn into glucose right away. But five hours later, they *do* digest into glucose and when they do, the 52 grams of carbohydrates found in each two ounce serving of pasta may hit your bloodstream with a nasty wallop. (Not to mention that you almost need a microscope to see a two ounce portion of pasta. Most people's idea of a portion of pasta is closer to six ounces—and 156 grams of carbohydrate!)

If you have pasta for dinner and don't see a peak by two hours after you have eaten, be sure to check your fasting blood sugar the next morning. You may see an unexpected blood sugar rise there which came from the pasta you ate the night before.

The people who can eat pasta or any kind of starch that resists digetsion without seeing a spike hours later are those who still have a robust second-phase insulin response. If you find a food containing a resistant starch that appears to work well for you, and if you don't detect a delayed spike hours later, you can conclude you still have a significant second phase insulin response left.

Sugar Alcohols and "Sugar Free" Foods

"Sugar free" foods are sold all over and promoted as being perfect for people with diabetes. The truth is that while they may not contain sucrose—table sugar—they are full of carbohydrates. Sugar free brownies or cookies are full of starchy flour. Sugar free ice cream is full of chemicals called "sugar alcohols" which have nothing to do with the kind of alcohol you drink.

Sugar alcohols are lab-created carbohydrates that may or may not break down into glucose in your body depending on whether you have the enzymes needed to digest them. If you don't, they won't raise your blood sugar, but they may give you horrible gas and diarrhea. If they don't give you the runs, they probably *will* raise your blood sugar because that means you can digest them, but they may do it so slowly that you may not see the blood sugar spike they cause if you only test one or two hours after eating them.

Again, as is the case with digestion-resistant starches, whether you can eat foods containing sugar alcohols without raising your blood sugar will have a lot to do with how much second-phase insulin response you have left.

Of all the sugar alcohols used in making "sugar free" products, maltitol is the one that is most likely to raise blood sugar. At least half of every gram of maltitol digests into glucose by the time three hours have passed since you have eaten it. So if a "sugar free" food seems to be kind to your blood sugar, try testing it an hour or two after you usually test. Erythritol is the one sugar alcohol that does not raise blood sugar, but it is rarely found in commercial "sugar free" products.

Dealing with Limited Blood Testing Supplies

In an ideal world, everyone would have all the testing supplies they need. But in real life blood sugar test strips are very expensive and many insurers sharply limit the number of strips people with Type 2 Diabetes can get each month.

Here are some strategies that can help you if your access to strips is limited:

- ❖ If you only have 50 strips to get you through a month, learn when your highest blood sugar is likely to occur after a meal. Do this by testing several meals one hour, one and a half hours, and two hours after eating. People who still have a strong second-phase insulin release will usually see a peak one hour after the end of their meals. Others may see a later peak. Once you know the time when you are likely peak, test at that time except when eating foods that are likely to be delayed, like pasta or food with sugar alcohols. Test those foods an hour later.

- ❖ Make the goal of your testing be to learn how many grams of carbohydrate you can tolerate in one meal. If you learn that 30 grams is your upper limit, use software and your food scale to find portions of other foods that will also clock in at 30 grams or less. Test one or two of these portions and if you see the result you expect you don't have to test every time you eat that amount of carbohydrate again.

- ❖ If you need more strips, consider the $35 you pay for a cheap meter and another 50 strips an investment in your health. It's far better to spend that $35 now, than to spend it on expensive doctor bills caused by complications you don't need to develop!

Avoid Becoming a Fanatic

Many people are so excited to learn that they can achieve normal blood sugars by cutting back on carbohydrates that they become zealots for low carbohydrate dieting. But it's important not to get too carried away with a "Carbs are Evil" mentality which makes it a matter of religious dogma never to eat those evil carbohydrates you've sworn off. Like all conversions this one tends to fade out in time, and, when it does, backsliding will follow. You need to control your blood sugar for the rest of your life, not for just as long as your enthusiasm lasts. So don't make carbohydrate restriction a religion. Treat it as a strategy which, when used in combination with many other strategies including medication, can give you normal blood sugars.

If you can be flexible and treat carbohydrate restriction as one of a variety of tools available to you to help you meet your blood sugar targets, you are more likely to be able to maintain excellent blood sugars for years to come.

Eliminate "Habit Carbs" and Concentrate on "Value Carbs"

When you start testing your favorite foods, you are likely to find that many of them contain far more carbohydrate than your body can handle. This may make you think that, thanks to diabetes, you will never again be able to eat any of your favorite foods. At first, when you are filled with relief at the discovery that you can still get normal blood sugars, despite diabetes, this may not seem like that big a deal. After all, most of are happy to give up donuts if it means we can also give up worrying about amputations or blindness.

But after a few weeks of devotion to your new lower carbohydrate diet you are likely to find yourself dreaming about eating the cakes or muffins or French fries you've sworn off. And as time goes on you may feel increasingly depressed that you can't eat any of these foods that used to mean so much to you.

Low carbohydrate enthusiasts will tell you that you shouldn't feel this way. Or they'll tell you that if you stick with the diet the feelings will go away. But after having stuck to a very low carbohydrate diet for over six years myself, I'm going to tell you that, while that approach may work for some people, for many of us who do not have a will of iron and a love of self-denial—or of a diet made up mostly of meats and healthy vegetables, it won't work.

Forbidding yourself a single bite of any carb-laden favorite food is a great way to program yourself for disaster. And the sad part is that most people with diabetes do not have to dedicate themselves to monk-like self-denial to get back their blood sugar control.

You *will* have to cut way back on the carbohydrates, but you can do this and still make room for foods that you have enjoyed all your life. Why? Because a quick look at your daily carbohydrate intake will often reveal that the bulk of the carbohydrates you are eating are what I call "habit carbs." These are the carbohydrates you eat without a second thought because they are there. Not because they taste good. Not because you couldn't live without them. Just because over the years you've gotten into the habit of eating them.

Here is a list of some prime "habit carbs."

❖ Cafeteria mashed potatoes made from powder

❖ Limp French fries

❖ Squashy hamburger buns

❖ Cardboard toast

❖ Cold home fries

❖ Stale boxed cookies

❖ Tasteless cellophane-wrapped pastries

❖ Rancid tortilla chips

❖ Waxy chemical-laden candy bars

How many of these flavorless, high carbohydrate foods have you been consuming every day just because they were there? Probably a lot more than you realize. The high carbohydrate foods that are really delightful to eat turn out, for most of us, to be few and far between. So before you lift that high carbohydrate fork-full to your mouth, ask yourself, "Is this food thrilling me?" If not, put it down. If it is, eat it, but pay attention to the flavor. Is it as delicious as you expected it to be? Does it even have much flavor? Would a piece of nice cheese or a few low carbohydrate nuts be as satisfying? The answers may surprise you!

Make a distinction between these "habit carbs" and what I call "value carbs," which are the carb-rich foods that really do deliver something worth indulging in from time to time. I'm not going to lie to you and tell you that you can eat them whenever you want. You can't. Not if you want to keep your blood sugar low enough to avoid developing diabetic complications. You aren't going to be able to eat them very often. But by using the strategies describe below, you should be able to eat enough of these foods to keep yourself from feeling deprived — and without derailing your diet or ruining your health.

Don't Create "Forbidden Fruits"

The key to long term success is to avoid endowing any food with the power that comes from making it forbidden.

If you've avoided eating bread for a couple of months, that humble roll in the restaurant bread basket may call out to you with an irresistible siren song. If you give in and eat it, with each bite you may find yourself feeling as if you are doing something incredibly sinful—the way you might have felt if you had eaten a whole box of chocolates in the past.

That feeling is the sign that you're heading for trouble. You've created a "forbidden fruit," and sooner or later that forbidden fruit is going to get you. You may declare that you will never again eat a roll—and then ruin your Thanksgiving holiday when you go to Aunt Glenda's and refuse to eat even a single one of her wonderful rolls that you have eaten every years since you were small, the ones that say, "This is our family Thanksgiving."

You may start to dream of rolls night after night. You may find yourself craving that roll all day long, feeling as if you could only to eat one roll you'd be happy, so incredibly happy. But of course diabetes has ruined your life, so you can't, which makes you totally depressed. You may start resenting family members or co-workers who have the gall to eat rolls in your presence and lecture them about how they are poisoning themselves with each bite they take.

Once that happens, it is only a matter of time until you end up crashing off the diet. You will eat that roll and then another and another. The resulting feeling of being out of control makes you wonder why you even bother trying to control your blood sugar. You listen to your doctor when he assures you that a 7.2% A1c is fine control and that there is no reason to be more stringent. You stop participating in diabetes support groups where you might encounter information that counters the denial you've sunk into. You pack on weight and tell yourself you don't care.

Not a pretty picture? Eh? But this is a scenario a lot of us have experienced. And that is why it is far better to make a bit of room in your diet for a roll every now and then and prevent these foods from building up a charge. When you give yourself permission to eat that object of desire every so often, you'll almost always find out that it doesn't taste anywhere near as good as you remembered it to. Then you'll be able to leave that food behind for the rest of the month without turning it into an object of obsession.

Just knowing that you can eat some specific off-plan food at some future time when you have scheduled an off-plan meal, makes it that much easier to say, "No thanks" to it the rest of the time and maintain your healthy blood sugar by eating the foods you can handle.

Provide Safety Valves

This is why many people with diabetes find it helpful to build safety valves into our diets. We don't call them "cheats" or say we were "bad" because those terms carry an emotional burden that is not helpful. We say we ate "off plan" because we know these high carbohydrate foods are not foods we can make an ongoing part of our daily food plan. When we eat them, they *do* raise our blood sugars too high. These foods include indulgences like cake, pastry, bagels, and waffles.

Because our goal is life-long blood sugar control, we accept that most of the time we will not be able to eat these foods. If we do, we will harm our health. But we also accept that we are human, so we schedule occasional meals where we can eat "off plan." We do this knowing that an occasional high blood sugar spike is not going to kill us as long as we are meeting our blood sugar targets the rest of the time. The "good enough" control we can adhere to year in and year out beats a few months of perfection followed by crashing off the diet entirely and ruining our health.

Whatever you do, aim to achieve your blood sugar targets most of the time to limit the likelihood that you will develop complications. If you go off plan, let it be no more than once a week. You are creating a safety valve for your food yearnings, not a bad habit!

Do the Diet Straight Before You Try Off-Plan Goodies

Changing your diet is mostly a matter of changing your habits. To succeed at eating in a way that doesn't raise your blood sugar you will have to break a lot of established habits and replace them with new ones. So when you start out working on blood sugar control, it's a good idea to eat only the foods that keep your blood sugar in the safe zone. Do this for long enough to establish new and healthier habits. This usually takes a couple months. Only when these new eating habits are firmly in place should you start working on the problem of how to deal with high carbohydrate temptations. But knowing that you will be able to work some of those beloved foods back into your plan eventually should help you get through this break-in period.

For your first three months let your meter be your guide. If your meter tells you a food raises your blood sugar over your target level, don't eat it again. Eat only the foods your blood sugar can tolerate.

Even the "healthy whole grains" and "low glycemic" foods dieticians are so enthusiastic about may turn out to raise your blood sugar too high.* They may work for people who are not diabetic—which includes most dietitians. But my diabetic body doesn't distinguish between oatmeal cereal and chocolate cake. Both have too many carbohydrates and both give me unacceptable blood sugars.

When you eat only the foods that don't raise your blood sugar, several things will happen. Within a few days you should stop feeling hungry. For the first time in years you may find yourself no longer dominated by food cravings and the relentless need to eat. The discovery that these cravings were not due to an emotional problem, but were caused entirely by the high blood sugar spikes you were experiencing, will be enormously reassuring.†

Another thing that will happen after you cut the sugar out of your diet for a few weeks, is that your sense of taste will change and you may be surprised to discover that vegetables taste much better than they used to. When you do eat something with sugar in it, you may find that the sweetness is almost unpleasant—far too much to your reeducated taste buds. These changes in your hunger level and sense of taste are what make it very easy for many people to stick with a low carbohydrate diet for a long time without feeling unduly deprived.

But if you attempt to add in off-plan foods before you are solidly on-plan, you may never really get to this point. Most people who crash on and off low carbohydrate diets do so because they don't eat at a carbohydrate intake level low enough to control their blood sugar long enough give them these benefits and motivate them to continue.

When you have finally gotten your blood sugar under control and started to enjoy the benefits, nothing horrible will happen if you make room for a small portion of some high carbohydrate treat every now and then. This may be heresy to some people committed to a low carbohydrate diet, but I am convinced it is the best way to ensure that

---

* The glycemic index was established by testing how foods raised the blood sugar of people who *did not have diabetes*. Their robust second-phase insulin releases could mop up slow digesting carbohydrates. But many foods a normal person can tolerate will not work for a person who has a slow or missing second-phase insulin release. And even among normal people it turns out that the glycemic index results are not reproducible. The food that appears to be low glycemic for one person is high glycemic for another.

† If you are still feeling unpleasantly hungry after cutting your carbohydrates dramatically, check that you are eating enough calories to support your metabolic needs. If you are, you may need a medication to counter your insulin resistance or you may need to talk to your doctor about using insulin because your own insulin production may not be enough to do the job. When you are controlling your carbohydrates and getting enough calories to provide your metabolic needs, *hunger is a symptom.*

bohydrate diet, but I am convinced it is the best way to ensure that this year's enthusiastic low carbohydrate dieter is a happy 5% Club member ten years from now.

How Often Can You Eat Off-Plan?

How often you have an off-plan food depends a lot on your dietary goals, how well you tolerate carbohydrates, and whether you are willing to exercise after eating. It also depends greatly on what medications you are taking for your diabetes.

Forty minutes of running, biking, weight lifting, or even brisk walking will burn off a lot of extra carbohydrates. So if you exercise regularly, try to eat your high carbohydrate treat before you head for the gym.

If you're trying to lose weight, you may have to keep off-plan treats few and far between until you near your weight goal.

You may want to schedule your off plan meal for a specific time— Saturday night, perhaps. Or you may decide you get one off plan meal a week. It's up to you.

Go with the Smallest Portion You Can Tolerate

When it is time to eat off plan, fill up with foods that are good to your blood sugar and then eat a small portion of the foods you find hard to handle.

If you have to eat a donut, eat one donut hole. Eat one slice of bread or one scoop of ice cream. Throw out half the fries before you eat the rest. Your goal is to eat enough to remember what the food tastes like and defuse it, and most importantly, to rediscover that few of these foods are anywhere near as good as you remembered them being.

Throw Away the Vocabulary of Self-Destructive Dieting

When you eat something with carbohydrates in it, don't think of it as a "cheat." Cheating is what you do when you're under the thumb of some authority figure—be it your 9th grade math teacher or the IRS. But *you* are the one in control of what you eat. So when you eat something that is off-plan, don't think of it as getting away with something. It is something you've decided to do for a very good reason.

Avoid getting into a power struggle with yourself. You'll always lose! If you keep eating things that were not what you had intended to eat, rather than beating yourself up, take it as a sign that your current food plan isn't working. Put some energy into figuring out *why* it isn't working. Are you having trouble finding foods in restaurants that don't raise your blood sugar? Maybe it's time to bring a lunch to work for a while or to find a new place to dine. Are you bored with what you have been eating? Google the Web for low carbohydrate recipes or join one of the big low carbohydrate discussion boards on the Web where hundreds of members exchange recipes and ideas for interesting things to eat. At **lowcarbfriends.com** or **forum.lowcarber.com** you will find many people who have done well eating a long-term low carbohydrate diet and who are eager to help you succeed.

Get your Nutrient Balance Right

If your problem is that your diet is making you hungry, try tweaking it. Are you eating too little food? Too little protein? Too much protein? Too little fat? Too few vegetables?

A healthy low carbohydrate diet should not be a low fat diet. Nor should it be a high protein diet. Most people who do best on a very low carbohydrate diet find they do best with 60-70% of their calories coming from fat and eating only as much protein as meets their nutritional needs.

Eating too much protein is a common mistake people make when they begin a low carbohydrate diet. You can learn what your real need for protein is while eating a low carbohydrate diet by visiting the Protein Need Calculator you will find on my Low Carb diet Web site at: **phlaunt.com/lowcarb/proteincalc1.php.**

After you cut way down on your carbohydrate intake, don't be afraid of fat. Though you may have been brainwashed that fat is evil, when you are eating very little carbohydrate, fat won't hurt you. Nor will it make you fat. I lost 18% of my startng body weight eating a diet that was 70% fat and maintained it for years afterwards on a high fat, low carbohydrate diet.

A long-term low carbohydrate diet should also be one filled with leafy greens like romaine lettuce and kale and with lots of the other low carbohydrate vegetables. Make sure you are eating a big green salad every day and several other servings of things like green beans, zucchini, or avocado. If you crave fruit, eat berries. If they are too expensive to buy fresh, buy them frozen and add them to one of the many low carbohydrate pancake recipes you can find. You'll find one on Page 179.

Another thing that can make you hungry is over-use of artificial sweeteners. A growing body of research suggests that artificial sweeteners increase appetite in both rodents and people. Cut out the diet soda and drink tea or seltzers for a week or two to see if that helps. MSG will make you hungry too. It occurs naturally in soy sauce and it is present in many packaged foods though you won't see it in the list of ingredients. Instead its presence is hidden by the use of alternative names like "hydrolyzed vegetable protein" or "natural flavoring." If you have eliminated sweeteners and MSG and are still feeling hungry, perhaps you need to eat slightly more carbohydrate than the amount you have settled on. Add a fiber cracker to each meal and see if that helps.

Whatever you do, keep the vocabulary of sin and guilt for the confessional. Your diet is not a moral issue, it's a metabolic one. Don't say, "I've been bad," say, "I went off plan." You're going to eat a lot of things in the years to come that will mess up your blood sugar. When you stumble, be kind to yourself. Dust yourself off and keep on going. Blood sugar control is a marathon, not a sprint.

When you slip up, recommit to doing the best you can do. If you hit your chosen blood sugar targets more often than not, you will end up a lot better off than if you don't try. The important thing is to keep at it, doing the best you can, and forgiving yourself when the best you can do isn't as good as you wish it were.

Know Your Limits

I've learned the hard way I can't eat *half* a blueberry muffin, so I don't try to use portion control for that particular food. I know blueberry muffins are trouble and I also know that I will eventually eat one. That's just how it is. Every blue moon or so I eat a blueberry muffin, experience the miserable high blood sugars that follow, and then remember why I don't eat muffins every day. What I don't do is fool myself that I can buy a muffin and only eat half. Everyone has a few foods that fall into this category. Treat them with caution!

Eat Off-Plan Foods Out of the House

I've also learned that if a big box of something full of carbohydrates is in the fridge, bad things are going to happen. So I try to eat my off-plan foods away from home. I eat my muffins or cookies at a coffee house. I have one slice of pizza at a pizzeria. I don't buy a box of muffins or a whole pizza and bring them home.

Getting this strategy to work requires that your whole family understand what's at stake. It took me a couple years of harping on what "complications" means, but by now, my family understands that if my blood sugar is too high, I'm damaging my body. They want to keep me around for a while and agree that I'm cuter with all my toes. So they understand that there are some foods that shouldn't be brought into the house—ever.

When other family members want to have treats at home, they are kind enough to buy things I don't like. For example, if someone wants Ben & Jerry's they buy the Chunky Monkey flavor I find revolting not the New York Fudge.

Over the years the nondiabetic members of my family learned that no one is doing themselves a favor scarfing down 300 grams of fast-acting carbohydrate every day—particularly not people with a family history of diabetes and heart disease! They also learned that there is no reason you have to eat bread and potatoes at every meal. The bread was in the drawer and if they wanted some they were free to get it, but it wasn't served with dinner out of habit.

Medications Can Help

I'm not a big fan of medications because there is just too much evidence that drug companies lie about side effects. I learned the hard way that some of these side effects are unpleasant and permanent, but I learned the hard way, too, that some of us—like, say, me—can't get normal blood sugars no matter how low our carbohydrate intake. For us, adding a diabetic drug or two to our daily regimen may be the only way we can get normal blood sugars.

Drugs I have found useful over the years include Metformin, Acarbose, and insulin. The new incretin drug, Byetta, helps some people make dramatic improvements in their blood sugar and their weight. Even after adding diabetes drugs to my daily regimen I've never been able to eat more than about 120 grams of carbohydrates a day, but after eating only 60 grams a day for many years, 120 grams of carbohydrates a day feels like a completely normal diet!

We will discuss the various drugs that may help you control your blood sugar in Chapter Eight. Just remember that all these diabetes drugs work best when you combine them with some level of carbohydrate restriction. How much restriction? After you've started a new medication, test your meals one and two hours after eating, and your blood sugar meter will tell you exactly how much carbohydrate you can eat with your new medication and still hit your blood sugar targets.

The Low Carbohydrate Diet is Safe

In case you are still being given out-of-date medical or nutritional advice by people who got their nutritional education back in the days when the now discredited low fat diet was believed to prevent heart disease, you should know that even the ultra-conservative American Diabetes Association now admits in its current practice guidelines that the low carbohydrate diet has been proven to be both safe and effective for people with diabetes.

A study which appeared in the Journal of the American Medical Association in 2007 found that an Atkins-style low carbohydrate diet not only caused double the weight loss of the low fat diet at the end of one year, but that it did not adversely affect cholesterol levels. This result, added to the finding of the Women's Health Initiative study, which represented $40 million dollars worth of high quality research, that *long-term adherence to a low fat diet does not prevent heart disease,* should lay to rest any last fears you might have about the impact of cutting carbohydrates on your health.

The findings of these studies are not news to those of us active on the Web who have seen our health improve on a low carbohydrate diet over the past decade, but they appear to have amazed the entire medical community. Still, many medical professionals continue to cling to their "Fat is Bad" religious belief no matter how many evidenced-based medical studies might contradict it. This is not surprising. It would be very hard for them to admit that they have spent their entire professional career giving people dietary advice that has actually worsened their health.

You will find a list of studies that support the safety of the low carbohydrate diet for people with diabetes in the Reference section on Page 183. Another excellent place to get information about the safety and efficacy of the low carbohydrate diet is Regina Wilshire's "Weight of the Evidence" blog: **weightoftheevidence.blogspot.com.**
Regina keeps up with the latest research and can help you understand just how poor the science is that is practiced by those who debunk it.

Chapter Eight
Diabetes Drugs

Though many people find that they can bring their blood sugar back into the normal range simply by limiting their carbohydrate intake, not everyone is willing or able to stick with a restrictive diet for the rest of their lives. That's why most doctors assume that dietary changes will not solve their patient's blood sugar problems and prescribe what are known as **oral antidiabetic drugs**.

These oral antidiabetic drugs include Metformin, Avandia, Actos, Glipizide, Starlix, Prandin, Byetta, and Januvia. Though they are called "antidiabetics" some of these drugs are occasionally prescribed for people whose blood sugars are prediabetic, since large studies have shown them to be effective for people with impaired glucose tolerance.

You may well be asking, if these drugs are so effective why should you bother with a complex and restrictive dietary regimen?

Effective, but Not Effective Enough

Unfortunately, the catch with these drugs lies in how you define "effective." Just as the American Diabetes Association's suggested blood sugar targets ignore the evidence pointing to the blood sugar levels at which damage occurs, the standard used by the FDA when it approves a drug as "effective for lowering blood sugar" falls well short of requiring that the drug bring blood sugar levels down to a level low enough to prevent complications.

So while an oral antidiabetic drug might be "effective" by the FDA definition of the term, this usually means only that the drug lowers the blood sugar of a person with a very high blood sugar slightly better than does taking no drug. A drug that lowers an A1c of 10% to 9.5% is considered effective, even though a person taking it still ends up with an average blood sugar of 261 mg/dl—a level high enough to guarantee complications.

When drugs are approved for use by people whose blood sugars are in the prediabetic range, they may only lower need to lower an OGTT result by 20 or 30 mg/dl. Since many people diagnosed with prediabetes have blood sugars that go up to 180 mg/dl or even 190 mg/dl after each meal, these drugs could still leave a prediabetic person with blood sugars that are well above 140 mg/dl for most of the day.

The limited power of these drugs to lower blood sugar is why oral antidiabetic drugs alone are not likely to bring your blood sugars back into the normal range. They are an add-on—not a substitute for dietary control. But here's the silver lining: if you restrict your carbohydrates and are still unable to get your blood sugars entirely back into the normal range, the addition of a well-chosen oral antidiabetic drug *may* be able to push your blood sugar levels down that last little bit you need to normalize them.

Now let's examine the commonly prescribed oral antidiabetic drugs to see what the lab research shows about what they do well, what they do poorly, and what you need to know before deciding whether they might be worth trying.

Metformin

Metformin is the generic name of the drug marketed as Glucophage. It was first discovered in the late 1950s. It has been used to control diabetic blood sugars in Europe since the 1970s and in the U.S. since the mid 1990s. It has also been the subject of a large study intended to see whether it could prevent impaired glucose tolerance from progressing to actual diabetes.

Why Doctors Prefer Metformin

The current American Diabetes Association practice recommendations state that Metformin should be the first drug prescribed for a person with Type 2 Diabetes. The reason for this is that, unlike other diabetes drugs, Metformin does not cause weight gain. Since many people with abnormal blood sugars already are overweight, doctors prefer to prescribe a drug that does not push weight in the wrong direction.

Metformin appears to reduce insulin resistance, and since many doctors believe that Type 2 is primarily caused by insulin resistance, this encourages them to prescribe it. Finally, there is evidence that Metformin has a protective effect on the circulatory system quite separate from its effect on blood sugars.

Metformin Inhibits the Liver's Production of Glucose

There is some scholarly debate about what exactly it is that Metformin really does, but most researchers agree that, for most people, Metformin keeps the liver from converting glycogen into glucose and dumping it into the bloodstream.

If you'll remember, the liver's tendency to dump additional glucose into the bloodstream can drive up blood sugar after a meal. The liver may also dump glucose in the bloodstream early in the morning when fasting insulin levels are low. So many people find that Metformin lowers their fasting blood sugar as well as their post-meal blood sugars.

Metformin May Stimulate Glucose Uptake in Muscles

Recent research suggests that Metformin may stimulate glucose uptake by muscles and inhibit glucose production by the liver by activating an enzyme, activated protein kinase (AMP), which is present in muscle, liver, and heart cells. This enzyme is usually activated when exercise has burnt off a muscle cell's energy stores. So Metformin may trick the muscles into behaving as if they have just exercised.

How Effective is Metformin?

How much does Metformin lower blood sugar? Not much, judging from the data published both in independent research studies and from the studies cited in the drug manufacturer's own official Prescribing Information.

In the manufacturer's Prescribing Information for Metformin ER, a chart reports the results of a study that showed that for 141 diabetic subjects put on Metformin, the average fasting plasma glucose dropped 53 mg/dl. However, the final fasting plasma glucose level in these subjects was still a whopping 189 mg/dl. No data is given in the Prescribing Information about the effect that Metformin had on their post-challenge blood sugar concentrations.

A study performed by researchers at the University of Texas in 1991, which did examine post-challenge blood sugar, gave glucose tolerance tests to 14 diabetic patients taking Metformin. The researchers found that Metformin reduced the average OGTT two hour result from 360 mg/dl to 306 mg/dl. This left the subjects with blood sugars that were still dangerously high. Metformin also reduced the subjects' fasting blood sugars from an average of 207 mg/dl to 158 mg/dl. Again this still left them with a toxic blood sugar level.

Another, larger, study which compared Metformin with Avandia put 100 newly diagnosed people with diabetes on Metformin and found that their average *fasting blood sugar* dropped from 223 mg/dl to 173 mg/dl, far above the level that might prevent complications. That study did not measure two hour OGTT values, but since the participants' A1cs dropped only to 7.1% which correlates with an average blood sugar of 175 mg/dl, they were most certainly still dangerously elevated.

Metformin Does Not Really Prevent Diabetes

The Diabetes Prevention Program Trials (DPPT) was a major study which examined whether prescribing Metformin could prevent people with prediabetes from progressing to full-fledged diabetes. Though the study was reported with headlines that said that Metformin could prevent the progression of impaired glucose tolerance to diabetes, examination of the study publications shows that, in fact, its effect was far more modest.

At the beginning of the DPPT study, the subjects' fasting blood sugars averaged 107 mg/dl and their average OGTT results were 165 mg/dl. Most were overweight—the average weight of the group, which was two thirds female, was 207 lbs.

During the first six months of taking Metformin, the subjects who were taking it saw their average fasting blood sugar drop by about 3 mg/dl, an insignificant decrease that did not help them achieve normal fasting glucose.

Over the rest of the four years of the study, their average fasting blood sugar rose back until it was almost identical to its starting level. The average A1c of the group followed a similar pattern, dropping by less than 1% during the first six months of the study to a level still far above normal and then rising over the next four years until it was very close to the 6.0% usually considered the A1c cutoff for diagnosing diabetes.

In their publications, the DPPT researchers chose not to include data about the change in the OGTT results of the study participants, though this data was collected. Given the rise in the A1c, the OGTT results probably showed a steady and depressing rise in post-challenge blood sugar levels.

Though their results made it clear that Metformin could not restore normal or even safe blood sugar levels, the researchers concluded that Metformin could prevent diabetes, since people in the Metformin intervention group became diabetic at a rate that was 31% less than those in the placebo group.

To understand why this isn't as impressive as it might sound, a subject in this study would have been considered "non-diabetic" if their fasting blood sugar was 125 mg/dl and would only have been called "diabetic" if that blood sugar was 126 mg/dl or more. So if the drug kept large numbers of people's fasting blood sugar in the 121-124 mg/dl range, it would be considered a success, though as we saw earlier, a fasting blood sugar that high just about guarantees that post-meal blood sugars are rising well into the over 200 mg/dl level which should be diagnosed as diabetic.

Once Off the Drug Many Participants Became Diabetic

That Metformin had made only a tiny downward shift in the blood sugar of many "nondiabetic" study subjects was made clear when a follow-up study found that within weeks of going off the drug, a quarter of the apparent risk reduction disappeared, because a surprising number of people who had been taking Metformin developed diabetic blood sugar levels as soon as they came off the drug. This suggested that the drug had no effect on the underlying process leading to diabetes. It had only slightly lowered the subjects' blood sugar levels while damage to their beta cells continued on unchecked.

Since the blood sugars of these subjects — who were instructed to eat a high carbohydrate, low fat diet — was almost certainly going well over 140 mg/dl after every meal and probably often reaching 200 mg/dl or higher, it should be no surprise that their underlying blood sugar control deteriorated. But unlike the original finding that Metformin appeared to prevent diabetes, this later finding received no play in the media and many doctors are still unaware of it.

So while taking Metformin might slow the progress of blood sugar deterioration by a very small amount, its use alone cannot bring blood sugars down to the normal level that might truly prevent beta cell dysfunction and organ damage.

Metformin Works Best When Blood Sugars are Very High

The reason Metformin's impact was so disappointing when it was given to people with prediabetes was made clear by some findings published by the University of Texas researchers: *Metformin works best when blood sugars are high and in people who are obese.* The UT researchers found that at normal blood sugar levels in people of normal weight

Metformin actually *decreased* rather than enhanced glucose uptake. This is in line with the finding that the primary way in which Metformin appears to work to lower fasting blood sugars is by limiting the production of glucose by the liver—a phenomenon more likely to occur in people whose fasting blood sugar is high—much closer to that 126 mg/dl ADA diabetes diagnostic level than to normal.

That this is true was made clear by the note in the published report on the DPPT study stating, "The effect of Metformin was less with a lower body mass index or a lower fasting glucose concentration than with higher values for those variables."

So the conclusion has to be that for people who are not obese and whose fasting blood sugar is still relatively under control, Metformin will only have a moderate effect.

There's No Research Data About the Effect of Combining Metformin with Carbohydrate Restriction

The foregoing might make you think Metformin isn't worth much. But despite what you just read, many people who discuss diabetes on the Web believe it to be the best and safest of the diabetes drugs. And despite the anemic study results, it seems to be far more helpful to people who limit their carbohydrate intake than it is to the people eating the high carbohydrate diet used in studies.

Metformin is also very helpful to people trying to lose weight. Messages posted on Web discussion groups suggest that people who have a lot of weight to lose whose weight loss has stalled out on a long-term low carbohydrate diet often start losing again when they add Metformin to their low carbohydrate diet regimen. Some people report that when they take Metformin while eating a low carbohydrate diet, they can eat slightly more carbohydrate per meal without spiking. Others report that it lowers their fasting blood sugar but not their post-meal numbers. The explanation for these differences probably lies in the differing underlying causes of their diabetes. Metformin may also make it easier to keep from gaining weight, too, especially for insulin resistant people who use injected insulin.

Metformin's Other Effects on the Body

Metformin appears to lower testosterone levels and for that reason it is often prescribed to women with Polycystic Ovary Syndrome (PCOS). It is possible that it has an impact on other hormones, and that may have something to do with its effects on weight.

Metformin has been reported to have a protective effect on the cardiovascular system independent of its effect on blood sugars.

How to Minimize Metformin's Gastric Side Effects

Because Metformin can cause gas or diarrhea, it's advisable to start out with a low dose and work up to an effective dose, which for most people is at least 1,000 mg a day. Lowering your carbohydrate intake while you take Metformin can help you avoid some of the more unpleasant gastric effects. It also helps to take Metformin on a full stomach. Avoid taking Metformin after taking a drug like Januvia or Byetta that delays digestion, as they can intensify the gastric side effects. Some people find that the extended release forms of Metformin—Metformin ER or Glucophage XR—produce fewer gastric side effects.

Another side effect that Metformin can produce, especially in people who have been taking it for a while, is a pain in the upper chest that may seem frighteningly like heart attack pain. Endocrinologists are aware of this side effect but many family doctors are not. When Metformin causes this kind of pain it seems to be due to irritation of the upper part of the stomach. Check with your doctor immediately if you experience such a pain to make sure that it is being caused by the drug, not something more serious!

If you do not respond strongly to Metformin, it may be worth asking your pharmacist to give you a version made by a different manufacturer. There appear to be differences in how well different generic brands work. Dr. Bernstein has observed that the Glucophage brand is more effective for his patients than the generics. I have found that the Teva brand of Metformin ER works best for me.

Can Metformin Cause Low Blood Sugar?

Metformin is not supposed to cause dangerous hypos. A very few people have found that it causes their blood sugar to drop low enough to make them uncomfortable. This may be because in some people it lowers blood sugars enough to cause the false hypos we discussed on Page 77.

Does Metformin Cause Lactic Acidosis?

Metformin is chemically similar to an earlier drug, Phenformin, which was taken off the market because it caused a fatal side effect, lactic acidosis. There is some debate about whether or not Metformin also causes this side effect.

One review of data from published studies suggests that the frequency with which lactic acidosis is found among people who take Metformin is the same as its incidence in populations not taking the drug. An epidemiological study in Canada found 10 cases of hospitalization for lactic acidosis in a population of 11,797 patients who had been prescribed Metformin.

The symptoms of lactic acidosis include malaise, muscle aches, and gastric distress that come on after a person has gotten over the initial problems associated with taking Metformin. It is possible that the incidence of lactic acidosis is higher than the statistics suggest because many doctors are aware that it can be a Metformin side effect and take patients off the drug immediately if they begin to exhibit any suggestive symptoms.

People with kidney damage, liver damage, or congestive heart failure should not take Metformin because they are more likely to developed lactic acidosis. Lactic Acidosis can also occur with dehydration in people who have otherwise normal kidney and liver function. People taking Metformin should discontinue taking it a few days before having a scheduled x-ray procedure that uses dye, since these procedures can affect kidney function and increase the risk of developing lactic acidosis. In an emergency where you need a scan requiring dye, doctors will usually give you the scan and instruct you to take no more Metformin for several days after the procedure.

Because of a fear that alcohol intake may enhance the risk of lactic acidosis, people taking Metformin are advised not to drink more than a very small amount of alcohol.

Metformin Depletes Vitamin B12 and Folate

Metformin has one more significant side effect. It may deplete Vitamin B12 and Folate and increases homocysteine, a blood chemical associated with increased heart attack risk. Because a very low carbohydrate diet may not provide enough of these important vitamins, B vitamin supplementation may be advisable for people on a very low carbohydrate diet who take this drug. If you have been taking Metformin for a while, you should ask your doctor to test your blood vitamin B12 level.

Low vitamin B12 is associated with increased neuropathy and exhaustion.

Acarbose: The Overlooked Diabetes Drug

Acarbose, sold under the brand name Precose, is a neglected but useful drug for controlling blood sugar. Like Metformin, it has been the subject of a large study to see if it can prevent subjects from progressing from prediabetes to full-fledged diabetes. Though it has long been prescribed in Europe, it is rarely used in the United States and many doctors are unaware of how helpful it can be to people with either diabetes or impaired glucose tolerance.

How Acarbose Works

Acarbose works by blocking alpha-glucosidase, the enzyme that chops starches and complex sugars into their component glucose molecules. When this enzyme is blocked, starches and complex sugars pass through the stomach and portions of the small intestine largely undigested rather than entering the bloodstream as glucose.

However, Acarbose is not that mythical substance so beloved by health scammers, the "starch blocker." That is because most of the starch and sugar whose digestion is temporarily blocked by Acarbose does, eventually, get broken down into glucose by the bacteria that live in the gut. The glucose contained in these foods then reaches the bloodstream. However, because the digestive process is slowed down, glucose is produced in dribs and drabs rather than in one big blood sugar-spiking dump.

How Much Improvement Does Acarbose Make in Blood Sugar?

The Prescribing Information provided by Bayer, the manufacturer of the Precose brand of Acarbose, reports that in clinical trials Precose lowered post-meal blood sugar numbers by 25 mg/dl to 83 mg/dl depending on dosage. At the most commonly prescribed dose, Precose caused a drop of 46 mg/dl. The same Prescribing Information insert also reports that in another study, subjects taking 100 mg of Precose over four months experienced an average drop in one hour post-meal numbers of 42.6 mg/dl.

Unfortunately, none of these studies reported the amount of carbohydrate that patients ate when they achieved these improvements. In one study published by Bayer the baseline one hour post-meal blood sugar of the subjects was a hefty 299.1 mg/dl, so even with the Precose, these study subjects were running blood sugars that were dangerously high. My guess is that they were eating the 60 to 100 grams of carbohydrate per meal routinely recommended by fat-phobic, diabetes-ignorant dietitians.

Adding Precose to Metformin only achieved an additional 31 mg/dl drop. However, unlike the case with Metformin alone, Precose appears to be equally effective for people who maintain healthy low blood sugar levels. In the past, when I used Precose along with a very low carbohydrate diet, I found that taking it allowed me to add an additional 15 to 20 grams of carbohydrate to my meal without seeing a dangerous spike.

Animal studies conducted throughout the 1990s suggested that even though this reduction in blood sugar was modest, Acarbose also decreased protein glycation and appeared to delay or prevent heart attacks and the other diabetic complications caused by elevated blood sugars.

Does Acarbose Prevent the Development of Diabetes?

To see if Acarbose could be used to prevent the progression of impaired glucose tolerance to diabetes, the multiple research centers that conducted the STOP-NIDDM Trial administered 100 mg of Acarbose three times a day to 714 subjects while giving another 715 subjects a placebo. At the end of three years a smaller percentage of the group taking Acarbose had developed diabetes than of the controls. The researchers concluded this meant Acarbose could significantly decrease the progress of IGT to diabetes. In addition, the people taking Acarbose appeared to have half as great a risk of cardiovascular events (heart attack, death, heart failure, stroke, or peripheral vascular disease) as controls. They also had less new cases of hypertension.

However, these conclusions were called into question by a review of the study which suggested that the results may have been manipulated by researchers connected to the drug's manufacturer.

Acarbose and a Low Carbohydrate Diet

There are no studies that look at what happens when people who are already controlling their carbohydrate intake use Acarbose to achieve healthy blood sugar targets. Anecdotal evidence suggests that when people eating a low carbohydrate diet use Acarbose to allow them to add an occasional high carbohydrate indulgence to their diet, it can be helpful.

However, Acarbose does not allow you to totally pig out. Eating more than an extra 20-30 grams of carbohydrate per meal with Acarbose may cause you to experience high blood sugar spikes three or four hours after eating, since that is when the starches and sugars will finally digest. The height of those spikes will depend on how much second-phase insulin release you have left.

Acarbose Does Not Block Simple Sugars

If you are using Acarbose, it is important to understand that it does not slow the digestion of simple sugars such as fructose or glucose because they do not require digestion but are absorbed from the stomach as soon as they are eaten.

Thus carbohydrates from corn syrup, maple syrup, or candies containing dextrose will go straight into your bloodstream, whether you have taken Acarbose or not. Acarbose works well with sucrose—table sugar—and starches like wheat flour, rice, and beans.

Dosing and Time to Take Effect

You should start out taking the lowest dose of Acarbose available and then work up. This will help you avoid gastric side effects. You take Acarbose with your first bite of food and it begins to work immediately.

Unlike other drugs, Acarbose does not get into your body in any significant amounts. It exerts its effect within the digestive tract and is not absorbed.

Gas—the Killer Side Effect of Acarbose

Fully 24% of the people assigned to the Acarbose group in the STOP-NIDDM study dropped out of the study long before it completed. There's a reason for that, and the reason is this: when undigested carbohydrate travels through your digestive tract the so-called friendly bacteria digest it. That kind of "digestion" also goes by the name of "fermentation" and one of its byproducts is gas.

This means that the more carbohydrates you eat with Acarbose, the more gas that will be produced in your gut. The resulting gas production can be intense enough to limit your social life—or motivate you to cut down on your carbohydrate intake very steeply, since you quickly learn to associate high carbohydrate dinners with hours of post-meal flatulence.

That, by the way, is why Bayer stopped marketing Precose brand

Acarbose in the US. Most Patients eating a typical high carbohydrate American diet were unable to tolerate it.

However, if you use Acarbose while eating at a more modest level of carbohydrate intake it can be useful.

Combining Acarbose and Metformin

Adding Acarbose to Metformin helps you achieve even better blood sugar control. However, I have also found it is better to use a lower dose of Metformin (500 mg/day) along with a lower dose of Acarbose (50 mg), since combining these drugs really ramps up the gas and gastric misery. Taking both drugs at a high dose simultaneously can result in acute stomach distress.

Drugs that Force the Pancreas to Overproduce Insulin

The drugs we've discussed up until now lower blood sugar by keeping glucose from going into the blood stream or encouraging the muscles to remove it from the blood. There is another group of oral antidiabetic drugs which lower blood sugar by forcing the beta cells to produce more insulin.

There are two families of these drugs: the sulfonylurea drugs, which include Glipizide (brand names Glucotrol and Glucotrol XL), Glyburide (Micronase, Glynase, and Diabeta), and Glimepiride (Amaryl) and the newer family of "glinide" drugs which include Stalix (Natalinide) and Prandin (Repaglinide).

The sulfonylurea drugs were the first oral diabetes drugs put into general use in the United states and the only oral diabetic drug available in the U.S. until the mid-1990s. They have been prescribed since the 1970s.

Too Much Insulin Can Lead to Dangerous Hypos

These drugs can lower post-meal blood sugars significantly. However, they do it at a cost. The sulfonylureas work by shutting a molecular gate in the beta cell which causes it to produce insulin whether or not there is any glucose in the bloodstream. This is quite different from the way a healthy beta cell functions. A healthy beta cell only secretes large amounts of insulin when blood sugar has risen over a certain threshold. The normal beta cell will also stop secreting insulin into the bloodstream as soon as blood sugar levels drop.

The sulfonylurea drugs only work if a person still has living beta cells, but in a person who still has some beta cells left, they can stimulate the production of surprising amounts of insulin. Because of this, they can occasionally cause low blood sugar attacks severe enough to cause unconsciousness or even death.

This is why people who take these drugs are encouraged to keep their carbohydrate consumption high and why many dietitians trained before the mid 1990s believe it is dangerous for people with diabetes who take oral drugs to let their blood sugar go lower than 100 mg/dl. While high carbohydrate consumption will help people taking these drugs avoid dangerous hypoglycemic episodes it may also ensure that their blood sugars are high enough to promote complications.

A single sulfonylurea pill may stay active in the body for eight hours. The "glinide" drugs are active for a shorter time, so when taken at meal time they are supposed to stimulate insulin production only when there is an elevated level of glucose in the bloodstream. Even so, users of these drugs report that they are still capable of causing hypos.

Both these families of insulin stimulating drugs can cause raging hunger which leads to weight gain.

More Insulin Means More Insulin Resistance

In addition, because both these families of drugs pour insulin into the bloodstream they will exacerbate insulin resistance rather than improve it. If you already are extremely insulin resistant and have the kind of diabetes characterized by higher than normal insulin levels rather than failing insulin secretion, the huge amounts of extra insulin that sulfonylurea drugs provoke may also stimulate overgrowth in your vascular system, since insulin is a growth hormone. Too much insulin may also promote the growth of cancers.

Some Sulfonylurea Drugs Increase the Risk of Heart Attack

The FDA-mandated Prescribing Information for Amaryl and other sulfonylurea drugs includes a black box warning stating that research on earlier sulfonylurea drugs has found that they may increase the risk of having a heart attack. A recently published study came up with the finding that the more sulfonylurea a person took, the higher the risk for a cardiac event" — i.e. a heart attack. This may be because some of these drugs not only stimulate the beta cells, but also stimulate a receptor in the heart. Prandin has also been found to be associated with more cardiac deaths.

A doctor commenting on this research recommends using only those insulin-stimulating drugs that have less effect on the receptor in the heart—Amaryl, Gliclizide, and Starlix. However, there is no research at present that appears to guarantee that they are safer. So they should be approached with caution.

Do Insulin Stimulating Drugs Cause Beta Cell Burnout?

There is some question about the wisdom of forcing already dysfunctional beta cells to produce yet more insulin. Dr. Richard K. Bernstein is a firm believer that these kinds of drugs cause beta cells to die and counsels people with diabetes to avoid them. However, there is little experimental data available to evaluate this possibility.

Some argue that UKPDS proved sulfonylurea drugs do not burn out beta cells since, in that study, those taking Metformin and sulfonylurea drugs experienced the same gradual decrease in blood sugar control over the years. But given the toxically high blood sugars subjects maintained in UKPDS, it is hard to know how much of their decline was due to any drug rather than exposure to very high blood sugars. There is no data on how sulfonylurea drugs affect people who maintain blood sugars low enough to avoid glucose toxicity.

More Insulin Means More Weight Gain

These drugs are associated with weight gain. This may be because they stimulate the relentless production of insulin. Some people believe that higher levels of circulating insulin cause weight gain. The weight gain may also be a result of the intense hunger people often experience when taking these drugs. That hunger may be due to the intense blood sugar fluctuations they cause or to some other, unknown, physiological effect. Whatever the cause, the hunger and weight gain associated with sulfonylurea drugs are a major reason why many people do not like taking them.

Sulfonylureas have another use besides stimulating the beta cells to produce insulin. They are also used as weed killers!

Byetta

Byetta is an injected drug which is surely the most hyped new diabetes drug to come along in years. Claims for it include that it produces massive weight loss without dieting, normalizes blood sugars, and regenerates beta cells.

Needless to say, the truth about it is more complex. Still, if you have Type 2 Diabetes, it is worth consideration.

What Byetta Does

Byetta is a substance that mimics a kind of hormone called an **incretin hormone.** Incretin hormones are produced by cells in the gut when they sense incoming food. One important incretin hormone, GLP-1, stimulates beta cells to secrete insulin, but only when the amount of glucose in the blood rises over a certain threshold.

Besides stimulating insulin production, GLP-1 regulates the stomach valves. When GLP-1 levels are high, the lower stomach valve does not open and a person will have a feeling of fullness after eating a small amount of food. GLP-1 may also influence how the brain experiences hunger.

Byetta is a molecule that is similar to naturally occurring GLP-1, however, unlike natural GLP-1 it does not break down swiftly, so its effects are longer lasting. The original molecule that formed the basis for designing Byetta was found in the spit of gila lizards, hence Byetta's nickname of "Lizard Spit."

Byetta is supposed to be injected twice a day. According to the Prescribing Information, its effect lasts for about two hours.

Why Byetta Promotes Weight Loss

When your stomach doesn't empty you feel full. Byetta shuts the stomach valve through which food passes into the intestines, sometimes for hours. This makes it physically impossible to overeat.

When you stop eating 100 grams of carbohydrate at each meal, your blood sugar drops. When you stop eating 1500 calories at each meal, your weight drops. Nothing magic here.

Byetta's effect on stomach emptying is probably the most significant thing it does for many of the people who find it helpful. That's what my endocrinologist has told me, and that's what many people using it report. It stops people from eating, and if overeating is contributing to their high blood sugars and weight gain, the drug will reduce both. Eating rocks would do the same thing, but not as safely.

Over time, this effect appears to wear off as does Byetta's effect on weight loss. This is clear from the studies cited in the official Byetta Prescribing Information.

Because of the delayed stomach emptying, people taking Byetta may also see wonderful numbers when they test their blood sugars after eating a high carbohydrate meal without realizing that their food has not yet been digested. If you take Byetta, you need to test your meals a few hours later than you'd usually test, to make sure that when the stomach finally does get around to releasing food into your gut you don't see a sudden spike.

People posting about their experiences with Byetta on the alt.support.diabetes newsgroup report that after using it they see the peaks they used to see at one and two hours occurring several hours later, at three and four hours. If those three and four hour peaks are over your blood sugar target, any improvements you are seeing at one and two hours after eating may be illusory.

Improved Glucose Response

Another thing that Byetta may do, at least in some people, is stimulate the pancreas to release more insulin when the food you've just eaten starts to raise your blood sugar. This is different from what the sulfonylurea drugs do because Byetta only stimulates insulin secretion when blood sugars have risen after a meal and the insulin secretion should stop when they drop. This means Byetta isn't likely to cause hypos the way that the sulfonylurea drugs do.

Byetta Works Very Well for a Small Subset of People

A small group of people taking Byetta report much more dramatic changes than the group as a whole, with some even experiencing complete normalization of their blood sugars.

These reports are anecdotal. The studies reported in the Byetta Prescribing Information showed that in a large group of people taking Byetta the average A1c dropped by only .5%. But I keep running into these "anecdotal" successes on the Web, and their enthusiasm is hard to ignore.

What are the Characteristics of These "High Responders"

Quite a few people who report the dramatic response to Byetta were in good control to start with. Unlike the people in the studies cited in the Prescribing Information, they started out with A1cs nearer 6% than 8%. That may be significant.

Several of them also are Jewish. This may also be significant, because we know that there is a defective gene found among people with

Type 2 Diabetes who are of Ashkenazi Jewish descent, a gene called HNF4-a, which has the effect of decreasing the postprandial secretion of insulin. The strong response of all the Jewish people I know who are on Byetta may be a sign that their diabetes is caused by a genetic failure to respond to rising blood sugars, and if that is so, Byetta may well correct this genetic defect.

Little Effect in Normal Responders

However, studies involving large groups of people taking Byetta make it clear that these dramatic responses occur only in a small subset of people. A manufacturer-supported study presented at the June 2007 ADA Scientific Session was reported very positively by the medical press who received a press release from its manufacturer titled, "BYETTA® Study Showed Sustained Blood Glucose Control Over Three Years in People with Type 2 Diabetes." But if you read the actual study, you find that what it really found was quite different. A more honest headline would have been, "Byetta Produced Damaging Blood Sugar Levels in 70% of those taking it." The press release the news coverage was based on bragged:

> After three years of BYETTA treatment, 46 percent of study participants achieved the American Diabetes Association's recommended target A1c of 7 percent and 30 percent of participants achieved an A1C of 6.5 percent.

So for the full 3 years of the study, 7 out of 10 of those taking Byetta had A1cs well over the American Association of Clinical Endocrinologist's target value—levels high enough to damage their organs. This study also found that Byetta produced trivial weight loss in most people taking it. Here's what the manufacturer's press release reports:

> Weight loss from baseline was progressive, with participants losing on average 11.68 +/ 0.88 lbs at three years. In addition, one in four patients lost an average of 28.66 lbs.

What this means is that one out of four people—the high responders we discussed earlier—did lose on average almost 10 pounds a year, three out of four people taking this expensive drug that did *not* control their blood sugar very, well lost an average of not quite *four pounds a year* over a three year period. In a population whose average weight was well over 200 lbs, this is not exactly miracle weight loss.

Does Byetta Regenerate Beta Cells?

The companies that make Byetta claim both in the media and when marketing the drug to doctors that Byetta regenerates beta cells. These claims rest on very sketchy data.

There is some mouse research showing that incretin hormones may regenerate beta cells. But when the question is asked, is this happening in people, the only data cited is data showing Byetta improving people's A1c, which doesn't mean that beta cells are regenerating, only that blood sugar control is improving. Since people on Byetta are eating a lot less of everything, including carbohydrates, the fact that they have slightly improved their A1cs does not necessarily mean that their beta cells are growing back.

Unfortunately, there is no way to examine the beta cells in the pancreas of a living person without destroying it. So we will not know if Byetta really grew new beta cells in humans until a lot of people taking it are dead. Because the FDA allows drug companies to make claims about the mechanisms by which their drugs work that are not well supported by peer-reviewed data, the drug companies will continue to claim that their drugs regenerate the pancreas based only on evidence of slightly improved A1cs.

Don't get taken in by this hype until it is much better supported. One finding that suggests to me that Byetta does *not* regenerate beta cells significantly is that in a follow-up study involving people originally involved in the Byetta drug acceptance trials who had been taking Byetta the longest, the blood sugar, after improving, reached a plateau and then started to deteriorate slightly again. The plateau reached was at a level where the patients still had diabetic blood sugars.

The Downside of Byetta

There are several major problems with Byetta. Some are well known, and the most troubling one is not.

Byetta Makes People Very Nauseated

About half the people taking Byetta get very nauseated. Some vomit. Some vomit a lot. This is caused by the way it shuts the lower stomach valve. Some people say this effect can be countered by wearing "Sea bands" which are an acupressure seasickness aid. Half of those taking it do not have this problem.

Byetta Does Not Work for Many People

If you scan through the many months worth of data at the Byetta blogs at **diabetes.blog.com** you'll see that there are quite a few people who do not get dramatic results from Byetta and another subset of people whose blood sugars worsen dramatically. What seems strange to me is how many people keep taking this expensive drug long after it seems clear it isn't having any effect.

Byetta Can Provoke Antibodies

A serious problem with Byetta may be that, like any injected protein, it provokes an antibody response, which in some cases can be very strong. When an antibody is produced, it latches onto the molecule that provoked it and keeps it from doing its job. If the molecule is the injected Byetta, that is one thing, but it is also possible that the antibodies Byetta produces may latch onto a person's own homemade incretin hormones and keep them from working, too.

If this is the case, the person might end up in worse shape than before they started the Byetta, because they have deactivated naturally occurring incretin hormones that might have been working until they took the drug.

The information in the Byetta Prescribing Information mentions that antibodies are produced and that in a small group of people a *lot* of antibodies are produced, but there is no further discussion on this. I have asked several knowledgeable endocrinologists about this problem but they say they only know what we both read in the Prescribing Information.

It is possible that production of these antibodies is the explanation for why some people have reported that their blood sugar gets far worse after they start Byetta. Others report that after taking it for a while, with success, their blood sugars shoot right back up when they stop taking it. This also casts some doubt on the claim that Byetta is regenerating beta cells. In all fairness, though, a few people who respond dramatically to Byetta report that they retain excellent blood sugars after losing a lot of weight and discontinuing the drug.

Byetta is Very Expensive

Unless you have very good insurance, the cost of Byetta may put it out of reach. It costs close to several hundred dollars a month. Many plans may limit your access to Byetta until you have tried other less expensive drugs.

Byetta May Cause Pancreatitis

On Oct 16, 2007, the FDA posted a warning about Byetta, saying that they had received 30 post-marketing reports of acute pancreatitis—a severe inflammation of the pancreas which can be fatal—some of which went on to kidney failure.

There is some controversy as to whether the incidence of pancreatitis found among people taking Byetta is higher than that of a similar population who is not taking the drug. Those representing the drug companies argue that all dieters and all obese people have a higher than normal rate of pancreatitis.

The FDA said doctors and patients taking Byetta need to be alert to the signs and symptoms of acute pancreatitis, which include persistent, severe abdominal pain that can radiate to the back and may be accompanied by nausea and vomiting. The incidence of this side effect appeared to rise after patients moved from the starting dose of 5 mc to the larger 10 mc dose.

Is Byetta for You?

Clearly, there has to be a cost/benefit analysis here. There are other effective treatments for diabetes and if you can get one of them to work for you, it might be better to wait another couple years to see what else we learn about Byetta's effects on the body. The drug is still very new, and most of the truly dangerous side effects of new medications do not show up until the drug has been taken by hundreds of thousands of people for a decade or more.

You are going to have diabetes for a long time, so if you can get good control by lowering your carbohydrate intake or using a proven drug like Metformin or insulin, there's no hurry. In another couple years we'll know much more about Byetta and if it does prove itself, you'll be able to use it safely. In addition, there is another drug very similar to Byetta currently undergoing testing which only requires injection once a week, rather than twice a day. If this drug proves to be safe, it might be much easier to use.

But because Byetta does have a transformative effect on some people with diabetes, it may be worth trying if you have not been able to control your diabetes with safer, proven therapies like cutting way back on your carbohydrate intake, and reducing your insulin resistance using exercise and metformin. The following guidelines should help you use it effectively with the least negative impact on your health.

❖ If you try Byetta for a month and your blood sugar gets worse, ask your doctor to help you find a medication that will work better for you. Even if Byetta is capable of regenerating beta cells, continual exposure to blood sugars over 200 mg/dl will eventually kill them off—along with the rest of the functional beta cells you had when you started the drug.

❖ If Byetta is having a strong impact on your hunger level and helping you to lose weight, but you are still seeing very high blood sugars, treat Byetta as a weight loss aid, but talk to your doctor about what you can do while you lose weight to better control your blood sugar.

❖ If you have not responded to drugs that stimulate insulin secretion like Amaryl or Prandin, it is not likely that you will get better blood sugar control with Byetta. You may be too insulin resistant for the amount of insulin secreted to make a difference, or your beta cells may be dead and no longer capable of secreting at all. In that case, you may need insulin supplementation rather than beta cell stimulation to control your blood sugar, though Byetta may help you with weight control.

❖ If you have not responded to Byetta, the other new oral incretin drug, Januvia, is not likely to do anything for you but lighten your wallet. Januvia raises naturally occurring GLP-1 rather than providing supplemental GLP-1 the way Byetta does. Byetta appears to be much stronger than Januvia. Many people who did respond to Byetta report disappointing results when they switch to Januvia.

Januvia

Januvia is a new drug which works on the incretin hormone system in a different way than Byetta does. While Byetta provides a synthetic version of GLP-1, Januvia allows GLP-1 secreted naturally by your body to rise to higher than normal levels. It does this by inhibiting the action of an enzyme called DPP-4. DPP-4 is a protease, which is a special kind of enzyme that destroys other biologically active compounds. DPP-4 does a lot of things, many of which have nothing to do with blood sugar. But one of its functions is to destroy naturally produced GLP-1 as well as another incretin hormone GIP (Gastric Inhibitory

Peptide). Like GLP-1, GIP stimulates insulin secretion when the concentration of glucose in the blood rises after a meal.

As is the case with Byetta, the studies cited in the Prescribing Information for Januvia suggest that it is only mildly effective. The study data showed that in a group of people whose average A1c was 8%, Januvia decreased the A1c of the group as a whole by a measly .6% — lowering it to a level significantly higher than even the dangerously high 7.0% A1c target recommended by the American Diabetes Association. The studies found that, when Januvia was added to Metformin or Avandia, it lowered the A1cs of about half of those taking the combination to 7.0%. The rest remained at dangerously high blood sugar levels.

However, anecdotal evidence posted by people taking Januvia suggests that, as is the case with Byetta, Januvia works very well for some people and not at all for others. Like Byetta, it appears to work best for people whose beta cells are able to respond to stimulation by sulfonylurea drugs, but it is weaker than Byetta and many people who responded well to Byetta did not find it effective when their doctors switched them to it.

Januvia is a pill, not an injection like Byetta, but it is, like Byetta, extremely expensive—almost $5 a tablet.

Januvia Side Effects

Because Januvia has only been on the market since late 2006, most information about its side effects comes from anedcotal reports from people who have taken it, including myself.

The most frequently reported Januvia side effects include:

❖ Heartburn

❖ Delayed stomach emptying and upper abdominal bloating after meals

❖ Constipation

❖ Sinus Headaches and cold symptoms which may increase in frequency and intensity the longer the drug is taken

❖ Changes in the inflammation response, for example increased inflammation at blood sugar testing sites or around cuts

How Long Until Januvia Takes Effect?

I was one of those for whom Januvia was very effective, and I saw an almost immediate improvement in blood sugars as soon as I started taking it. By two weeks the blood sugar lowering effect was only a bit stronger than when I started it, though my feeling of well-being had increased significantly. When I stopped Januvia, it took exactly one week for its effect on my blood sugars to fade out completely.

Many people report seeing no effects at all after taking it, but are encouraged by their doctors to continue anyway, because doctors have been told by drug company salespeople that, like Byetta, Januvia will regenerate their beta cells.

This claim is far from proven, but we know for certain that glucose toxicity—the poisoning effect high blood sugars have on beta cells—are likely to kill any newly regenerated beta cells were they to exist. So if you see rapidly escalating blood sugars after taking Januvia for more than a month, insist that your doctor help you find a more effective way of controlling your blood sugar.

Januvia's Impact on Inflammation

After I'd been taking Januvia for a few weeks I cut myself while cooking. It was just a little cut, but it seemed to take forever to heal. At the same time I noticed that I was getting sore spots on my fingers where I was testing my blood sugar. This really was unusual. I'd been testing 6-8 times a day while on insulin and my fingers never hurt. Suddenly they were getting red and sore.

I posted about this experience on the Januvia blog maintained by The Diabetes Monitor. Almost immediately someone chimed in saying that they had also noticed slow wound healing which went away when they stopped the Januvia. A nurse reported to me by email that she noticed very slow healing after gum surgery while taking Januvia which appeared to improve after she stopped the drug. Another person taking Januvia reported significant white blood count changes after starting Januvia. Yet another person reported coming down with pinkeye after starting Januvia. Yes, these were anecdotal reports. But given that scientists know that DPP-4 plays an important role in regulating the immune system and given that the approval process for Januvia did *not* include any studies about the impact of inhibiting DPP-4 on the immune system, they were troubling.

A study which measured the concentrations of DPP-4 in both mice with an induced autoimmune arthritis and people with rheumatoid arthritis found that *the lower the DPP-4 levels, the higher the degree of inflammation.*

The manufacturer's Prescribing Information for Januvia does not discuss changes in the immune system caused by the drug except to say that,

> Across clinical studies, a small increase in white blood cell count (approximately 200 cells/microL difference in WBC vs. placebo; mean baseline WBC approximately 6600 cells/microL) was observed due to an increase in neutrophils. This observation was seen in most but not all studies. This change in laboratory parameters is not considered to be clinically relevant.

A helpful email from a leading DPP-4 researcher who sent me some publications about Januvia that are not available on the Web, suggests that Januvia does indeed cause more persistent inflammation during the healing of wounds. This is because another function of DPP-4 is to cut up and get rid of cytokines, which are the substances that cause inflammation. So when DPP-4 is inhibited, the cytokines that cause inflammation rise to higher levels.

Rash and Skin Side Effects

People taking Januvia sent me two anecdotal reports of allergic rashes during the first six months the drug was on the market. In October of 2007, six months later, the manufacturer added the following information to their FDA-approved Prescribing Information: "These reactions include anaphylaxis, angioedema and exfoliative skin conditions including Stevens-Johnson syndrome."

This confirms that swelling, rashes, and peeling skin may indeed be side effects of Januvia. Stevens-Johnson syndrome is a serious immune-system related problem where large portions of skin may separate from the body. It can be fatal. So if you experience a rash while using Januvia, take it seriously and do not let your doctor tell you that Januvia doesn't cause a rash. It is very important to understand that Januvia inhibits the action of a vital component of the immune system in ways that are *not* fully understood.

I have also received a report of tongue swelling associated with Januvia.

Could Januvia Promote Cancer?

In the course of reading up about the other functions of DPP-4 in the body, I discovered something that raised a very serious concern about what Januvia's long term side effects might be.

It turns out that the suppression of DPP-4 appears to be involved in the transformation of melanocytes and prostate cells into malignant cancer cells. As one study states, "downregulation of DPPIV [i.e. DPP-4] is an important early event in the pathogenesis of melanoma." The report continues, "Malignant cells, including melanomas and carcinomas, frequently lose or alter DPPIV cell surface expression. Loss of DPPIV expression occurs during melanoma progression at a stage where transformed melanocytes become independent of exogenous growth factors for survival." [i.e. the cells stop expressing DPPIV when they start to turn into viable tumor cells.]

Furthermore, "Reexpressing DPPIV in melanoma cells at or below levels expressed by normal melanocytes induced a profound change in phenotype that was characteristic of normal melanocytes." In short, turning DPP-4 expression back on stopped the cells from behaving like cancer cells.

A similar effect was observed with ovarian cancer cells. The researchers state, "We investigated the correlation between DPPIV expression and progressive potential in ovarian carcinoma. We demonstrated that ovarian carcinoma *cell lines with higher DPPIV expression were less invasive.* [Emphasis mine]"

As I'm a melanoma survivor, this information convinced me to stop taking Januvia immediately despite its excellent effect on my blood sugars. I cannot afford to play around with any chemical that might be hastening the process by which rogue melanocytes become malignant!

Please note that I am not saying that Januvia causes cancer. Given the complete lack of research into the effect of long-term suppression of DPP-4 on the growth of pre-existing melanoma, prostate, and ovarian cancer cells in the body, we have no way of knowing whether it does or not. All we know is that Januvia inhibits an enzyme that is related in some way to the transformation of normal cells into cancer cells.

We also know that in a group of about 2,000 people who took the drug for the two year period that the Januvia approval trials lasted there was not an observable increase in cancers. Given that cancers like melanoma or ovarian cancer may develop very slowly before becoming malignant—mine developed over a period of about seven years—and that the incidence of melanoma is low enough that a significant increase in melanoma cases might not be seen in a group as small as the one involved in this test, this does not mean much.

We'll only know for sure if taking Januvia results in people getting more malignant cancers after many hundreds of thousands of people have taken the drug for a decade or more. Even then, any increase in the number or virulence of these cancers may never be connected to the drug. The only way the FDA will learn about the Januvia/cancer connection is through doctors reporting the connection using the poorly designed aftermarket reporting system. Since most doctors have no idea that there is any relationship between DPP-4 and melanoma, they are very unlikely to connect Januvia with new cases of melanoma or ovarian cancer that develop in people who have been taking Januvia for four or five years.

So if you are a melanoma or ovarian cancer survivor, or for that matter, any kind of cancer survivor who may still have malignant cells in your body, Januvia looks like a poor choice no matter what its effect on your blood sugar. You don't want to gamble with anything that inhibits the mechanism your body may be using to keep cancerous cells under control.

If you are a cancer survivor and want to investigate the effect of an incretin-based drug on your blood sugar, Byetta would be a better choice. It has no effect on DPP-4, but is simply an artificial form of the naturally occurring gut hormone, GLP-1.

Avandia and Actos

Avandia and Actos are two very similar drugs that are part of the family of thiazolidinediones (TZD). They are a relatively new class of oral antidiabetic drugs which were developed during the 1990s. Three of these drugs began their careers by showing great promise in the treatment of insulin resistance, and hopes were raised by preliminary research that they might be able to rescue beta cells.

Unfortunately, over time all three were found to cause life-threatening side effects, the risk of which was far greater than the benefit these drugs provided. The hope that they might rescue failing beta cells also proved to be a mirage.

Rezulin, the first of these drugs and the one that endocrinologists tell me was by far the most effective, was withdrawn after it was found to cause fatal liver failure in a small but significant number of patients.

Avandia (Rosiglitazone) and Actos (Pioglitazone) came to market in the late 1990s with the promise that they did not cause liver failure — though post-marketing reports later discovered that this is not entirely true. There are reports of liver failure associated with these drugs.

But it took almost a decade for the real problems with these drugs to surface. One reason for the delay was that the manufacturer of one of the drugs intimidated whistleblowers in the medical community who called attention to their dangers.

What These Drugs Do

These drugs work by decreasing insulin resistance. This sounds exciting until you learn that they do this by causing the formation of new fat cells, primarily on the arms, thighs, and butt, into which insulin pushes excess glucose taken from the bloodstream.

Like the other, safer, oral diabetes drugs discussed earlier in this chapter, the manufacturer's own official Prescribing Information makes it clear that whatever it is that they do, the TZDs produce only a modest change in blood sugar and insulin levels, though some research suggests they produce slightly better blood sugars than Metformin does.

Studies funded by its manufacturer suggest that Actos may improve endothelial dysfunction — which might in turn lower the risk of vascular complications. They also suggested it might decrease the kind of inflammation associated with coronary artery disease and improve high blood pressure.

Beta Cell Rest Proved to be a Myth

Other research showed that Actos preserved the beta cell islet structure in two strains of diabetic mice whose diabetes was caused by damaging a specific gene. This raised hope that it might do something similar for people. The premise that TZDs could rejuvenate beta cells was promoted so effectively by drug company sales people that many patients now take these drugs in the belief they are reviving those cells, even when they experience serious side effects and see little effect on their blood sugars.

But the hope that TZD drugs could rejuvenate beta cells was dashed by the publication in 2007 of results from a large study of Avandia. The study, called DREAM, went on to become a nightmare for those taking the drug. DREAM had initially appeared to show that taking Avandia could prevent the onset of diabetes — but the follow-up found that as soon as the drug was stopped, people developed diabetes at the same rate as if they hadn't taken the drug. This makes it crystal clear that the claim that these drugs help the beta cells heal themselves is not true. Had beta cells been rejuvenated, blood sugar response would have been improved after the drug was discontinued.

Avandia Causes Heart Attacks

That was just the beginning of the bad news that came out of the DREAM follow-up study. The study had been funded by Avandia's manufacturer, GlaxoSmithWellcome, in the hope that it would prove that Avandia would prevent heart disease. Instead it found the opposite.

The DREAM study found that patients who took Avandia had 66% percent more heart attacks, 39% more strokes, and 20% more deaths from cardiovascular related problems than those who did not.

Then the news came out that in 1999 Glaxo had silenced an early critic of Avandia who had uncovered evidence pointing to Avandia's connection with heart problems. The drug company had shut him up by threatening to bring an expensive law suit against the critic's university. The threat was effective and the scientist did not make public the information he had about Avandia's possible role in causing heart attacks. Only in 2007 did FDA drug reviewers finally publish a report confirming that patients taking Avandia are more likely to suffer and die from heart problems than those taking Actos.

Avandia is Most Dangerous when Combined with Insulin

The most serious heart problems associated with Avandia appear to occur when patients combine Avandia with insulin, which is a combination that Glaxo had been pushing as part of a three drug strategy including Metformin, which it claimed avoided weight gain. The combination with insulin increases the incidence of heart failure, which is a weakening of the heart muscle that leads, inexorably, to death.

The 2007 FDA report about Avandia suggested that Actos is safer, and indeed, many doctors had started to switch patients to Actos after the reports of Avandia's relationship to heart attack were made public. But given that the mechanism by which the two drugs work is very similar, the safety of Actos is also questionable.

Indeed, only a day after the FDA report came out, another study was published in the journal, *Diabetes Care*, suggesting both Avandia and Actos cause heart failure in younger patients with no previous history of heart failure. The analysis in *Diabetes Care* projected that one in every 50 patients who takes Avandia or Actos over a 26 month period would be hospitalized for heart failure. The researchers found that one fourth of cases occur in people younger than 60. Normally heart failure tends to affect older people.

The Most Recent Research Suggests Actos is Not Very Effective

A meta-study published in October of 2006 which analyzed the results of 22 randomized clinical trials involving 6,200 patients with Type 2 Diabetes who took Actos concluded that,

> Our results showed that published scientific studies of at least 24 weeks of pioglitazone [Actos] treatment in people with Type 2 Diabetes mellitus did not provide convincing evidence that patient-oriented outcomes like mortality, morbidity, adverse effects and health-related quality of life are positively influenced by this drug. Until new evidence becomes available, the benefit-risk ratio of pioglitazone [Actos] therapy in Type 2 Diabetes mellitus remains unclear.

According to Dr Richter, the author of this study, not only did the review demonstrate no clear-cut benefit to using Actos, but it also showed an increased occurrence of edema [water swelling] and heart failure—including heart failure requiring hospital admission—among patients taking the drug.

Actos and Avandia Grow New and Permanent Fat Cells

Even without these very disturbing findings, there is another big problem with Actos and Avandia. They pack on weight.

It has long been known that all the drugs in the thiazolidinedione family cause weight gain. Because they also cause the water retention and swelling that now are linked with heart failure, it was first believed that this weight gain attributed to these drugs was caused solely by water retention.

When it was later determined that *real fat* was being deposited on the bodies of those taking it, the drug companies spun this information by claiming that in people taking the drug the hip/waist ratio had changed. They suggested this might be because abdominal fat—the kind known to correlate with insulin resistance—was decreasing, which would be a good thing.

However, when a group of researchers randomized a group of

nondiabetic insulin resistant volunteers to either diet and exercise or Actos, they discovered that d*ecrease in waist hip ratio that study subjects experienced while taking Actos was due to the increase in their hips, not a decrease in their waist.*

The study found that Actos was causing an increase in the number of fat cells accumulating in what was euphemistically called "the lower body depot" in an area most of us would probably recognize better when called by its common name: the butt.

This is troubling, because once you add new fat cells they do not go away even when you diet.

Calorie Restriction and Exercise Work Better than TZDs

It is even more troubling to learn that the blood sugar improvements Actos made in the study subjects taking it could have been achieved without adding new fat cells to their butts. The group of insulin resistant volunteers in the study just cited who took *no drug* but cut 500 calories a day from their diet and exercised for 45 minutes a day achieved far better improvements in their fasting insulin levels, their fasting triglyceride levels, and their total cholesterol than did the Actos group—while losing weight from both their waists and their "lower body depot."

Other Serious Side Effects of Actos and Avandia

Macular Edema

Another dangerous side effect that has been associated with both TZD drugs is macular edema—swelling in the retina which can lead to blindness. This swelling does not always resolve when the drug is discontinued.

Liver Toxicity

Despite the original claim that they were not toxic to the liver, there have been a few reports of liver disease occurring in patients taking these drugs. While it does appear they are less damaging than Rezulin, they do raise liver enzymes. This is usually interpreted to mean that liver damage is occurring. Experts suggest that monitoring liver enzymes may not be enough to prevent damage.

Bone loss with TZD

Several studies have shown that elderly women taking Avandia and Actos are likely to suffer more bone loss leading to fractures than would be expected. This finding was reinforced by another study by Dr. Steven Kahn published in the *New England Journal of Medicine*. It compared Avandia to Metformin and Glyburide and found twice as many bone fractures in the group of patients taking Avandia. Actos has also been found to cause a doubling of fractures in a group of patients taking it for a relatively short period, less than 3 years.

The mechanism by which these drugs cause fractures appears to be that they create new fat cells by stimulating the cells that are supposed to turn into new bone cells in such a way that they turn into baby fat cells instead. Over time the bones become porous as they have been deprived of the new bone cells they need for repair.

The studies that found increased osteoporosis and broken bones in people who had used these drugs were conducted over fairly short periods. This is probably why they only noticed the bone problem in older women. Older women have less bone mass than younger women or men have, so any deterioration in their bone would be more obvious. Over time bone brittleness could become a problem in all people taking this class of drugs.

How Can You Stay Safe with New Drugs?

After reading the above you may well be wondering if it is safe to take any drug. The answer is a qualified maybe.

After a drug is approved, it usually takes many years for its dangerous long-term side effects to become known. So it is wise to resist the impulse to take any brand new drug. Wait until it has been on the market for a few years. Even then, proceed with caution. Avandia was on the market for almost twelve years before its ability to cause heart attacks, heart failure, and osteoporosis became generally known.

Doctors get most of their information about new drugs from salespeople sent out by the drug companies. Most studies of these drugs are done by the drug companies too. So there is very little unbiased information available about the safety of any new drug. Even worse, once the drug is approved by the FDA, drug companies have little incentive to do any research that will turn up bad news about their products.

Here are a few guidelines to help you stay safe:

❖ Before you take *any* new drug, download the "Prescribing Information" for that drug. The "Prescribing Information" is a legal document required by the FDA. It has to be kept up-to-date. It is the "label" you see mentioned in articles about the drug. Your pharmacist can also give you copies of the latest version of the Prescribing Information.

❖ The Prescribing Information will list all the known serious side effects of a drug. Even though the FDA usually does no more than issue a slap on the wrist when a serious side effect is discovered, it does make the drug company mention the side effect in the Prescribing Information.

❖ Make sure you understand the Prescribing Information. If your medical knowledge isn't good enough to understand the wording, do not be shy about calling up your doctor or pharmacist and asking them to interpret it for you. The information contained in the Prescribing Information may be as big a surprise to your doctor as it is to you.

❖ If a drug may produce serious side effects, ask your doctor whether there are tests that can spot these side effects early enough to prevent permanent damage. Then make sure your doctor does those tests. Even here, there is the concern that the drug company may have told your doctor that certain tests can guarantee safety when this is not true. With Rezulin, by the time liver enzyme tests warned of liver damage, it was too late to reverse the damage for some of the victims who then died of liver failure.

❖ Ask your doctor if there is an older, better understood drug or other healing strategy that could be used instead of the newer drug.

❖ If your doctor claims that a new drug does something really important no other drug does, such as grow new beta cells, and tells you that is why you should take it, check out the actual research on the **bloodsugar101.com** Web site.

All this sounds like a lot of work, and it is. But since your doctor is too busy to do it, you will have to. It is *your* body that will pay the price if you take a toxic drug.

Chapter Nine
Insulin

Nothing raises as much fear in the minds of most people with Type 2 Diabetes as the thought of having to go on insulin. This is a tragedy, because, of all the medications available to diabetics, insulin is the only one capable of not just lowering, but of normalizing, their blood sugar.

There are a lot of things about diabetes that should be terrifying: blindness, amputation, kidney failure, impotence, and, worst of all, the very high likelihood of dying, much too young, of a heart attack. All these are caused by prolonged exposure to high blood sugars, including blood sugars reaching levels that many doctors consider too low to be worthy of any drug treatment at all.

Insulin can prevent all these terrible things from happening. So why waste your fear on it?

We will look now at what it is that people with diabetes fear about insulin and examine why their fears are groundless.

Needles

Needles scare a lot of us, because the needle doctors use to give us immunization shots or to draw blood hurt. Fortunately, insulin needles are much thinner and do not. It comes as a pleasant surprise to many people with Type 2s Diabetes to learn that the ultra-thin short needles used for injecting insulin are even less painful than the lancets they use to test their blood sugar. Most of the time these needles are so painless that when you inject you may have to take a look to see if you actually have penetrated the skin, because you can't feel the needle!

Some family doctors may be unaware that there are newer thinner, shorter needles available for insulin and instead prescribe long thick gauge needles. These can be painful. If you were first prescribed insulin at a hospital, you probably were given shots with a thick needle, too. The reason for this is that there is always the possibility that the hospital staff members who give injections might be exposed to blood borne diseases. So hospitals mandate that staff use specially capped needles that have been designed to make it less likely they will stick themselves. These needles only come in thicker gauges.

Blood borne disease is not a problem for you when you are injecting yourself, so insist that your doctor prescribe the thinnest, shortest needle possible. Ask a pharmacist to recommend the best needle for you, if your doctor does not have information about needle gauges.

The second important thing to know about injecting insulin is that when you first start out, and are panicking at the idea of giving yourself a shot, it helps to "throw" the syringe at your injection site the way you'd throw a dart, holding the syringe with three fingers and tossing it at your target—usually belly fat—starting from 6 or 7 inches away. The swift motion of the needle completely eliminates any sting or feeling of the needle going in and will help you get over your natural anxiety about injecting yourself. Once you are used to injecting, you can just push the needle in.

Fear of Hypos

The other major fear that keeps people with Type 2 Diabetes from using insulin is the fear that they will have dangerous or even fatal hypos—low blood sugar attacks caused by taking too much insulin. We've all seen the movies where someone goes into "insulin shock" and nearly dies.

Hypos are a possibility, but no more so than they are with sulfonylurea drugs like Amaryl. The advantage of injecting insulin is that you have a lot more control over the *dose* of insulin you get than you do with an insulin-stimulating pill. So if you take some time to study how to use insulin you should be able to avoid serious hypos completely. It does take some study. Using insulin is more work than swallowing a pill. But unlike most pills, *insulin works*! If you get the dose right and keep your carbohydrates under control, insulin can lower any blood sugar to a safe and normal level.

Once on Insulin Always on Insulin?

Another reason people fear insulin is that they may have heard that once you start insulin you will never be able to stop using it. Observing what happened to their diabetic relatives, they may also conclude that once a person starts insulin it is only a matter of time until they suffer blindness, amputation, and kidney failure.

This misunderstanding is caused by the fact that in the past many doctors delayed giving patients insulin until long after they needed it. So by the time they started it, they were contending with decades of damage produced by exposure to high blood sugars.

Up-to-date doctors now know that if they intervene early and use insulin to bring down extremely high blood sugars soon after diagnosis, people with Type 2 Diabetes are more likely to regain excellent control and be able to stop using insulin. Very high blood sugars greatly increase insulin resistance and using insulin to lower them can improve it.

Insulin Must be Tailored to Your Own Metabolism

The most important thing to understand about insulin is that the dose that works for you is going to be different from the dose that works for someone else, because your physiology is different. Because of this, when you first start using insulin your doctor should put you on a low dose and ask you to record your blood sugars. Then he should slowly raise the dose in small increments until you reach the levels where your blood sugars should be. If your doctor isn't willing to work with you to pick a starting dose and then work towards getting it just right, so that your blood sugars become normal, you probably need to find a better doctor or a Certified Diabetes Educator who can help you do this.

Unfortunately, all too often doctors give people with Type 2 Diabetes generic doses of insulin. These doses may be too high. If that is the case, the patient will have to eat a lot of carbohydrate to keep from having hypos. The combination of a lot of insulin and a lot of carbohydrate usually results in steep blood sugar fluctuations. Those fluctuations cause hunger, overeating, and weight gain. If the generic dose is too small, blood sugars drop but remain high enough to damage health and because blood sugars are still surging and dropping, you may become very hungry and gain weight. Only when your doctor or educator takes the time to teach you how to adjust your blood sugars so you can "walk up" to the correct dose will you end up with the kind of blood sugars you want. When you have found that right dose, your blood sugars should stay relatively flat and you should not be hungry.

It goes beyond the scope of this book to explain insulin dosing to you in detail, but you can learn what you need to know from a CDE or a good doctor. Supplement that with what you can read in the books *Dr. Bernstein's Diabetes Solution*, by Dr. Richard K. Bernstein or *Think Like a Pancreas*, by Gary Scheiner. *Using Insulin* by John Walsh is another book that is often recommended.

The Two Different Kinds of Insulin

There are two different kinds of insulin doctors can prescribe: basal insulin and fast-acting insulin. Most people with Type 2s Diabetes, when they go on insulin, are put on a **basal insulin**.

It is important to understand what a basal insulin does — and what it does not do. *Basal insulins only affect your fasting blood sugar level.* They are not able to lower the high post-meal blood sugars you get after eating a meal filled with carbohydrates.

Using Basal Insulin

Basal insulin attempts to mimic the basal insulin secretion we discussed in Chapter One. Basal insulin, once injected, is slowly absorbed into the body over a long period of time. It provides a steady background dose of insulin. A single injection of Lantus usually lasts from 18-24 hours. An injection of Levemir lasts 12 hours or more depending on dose size. Both are newer, more expensive basal insulins. They provide a steady dribble of insulin into your bloodstream.

NPH is an older, cheaper basal insulin that is not as steady in its action as these newer insulins. It is absorbed erratically, so people using NPH may experience insulin hitting their bloodstream at unpredictable times. This makes it tougher to use. The tendency of this older insulin to cause sudden drops in blood sugar is one reason why older doctors worry so much about hypos. The newer basal insulins are much more predictable in their effect. If you get your Lantus or Levemir dose set properly, you should not have to worry about hypos.

But it is important to understand that *basal insulin does not counteract the blood sugar spikes caused by eating carbohydrates.* When dosed properly, basal insulin should only affect your fasting and pre-meal blood sugars. It should have little or no impact on your post-meal readings.

But by now you understand that high blood sugars after meals are the major cause of organ damage. And knowing that, you should be able to see what the problem is with using an insulin regimen that only involves basal insulin: It doesn't lower post-meal spikes. This is why all too many people with Type 2 Diabetes who are "on insulin" still have A1cs over 7.0% — often a lot over 7.0%.

Fast-Acting Insulin

Fast-acting insulin is injected to cover a specific meal. Humalog, Novolog, Apidra, Humulin R, and Novolin R are all brand names of fast-acting insulins. Typically these insulins begin to work within 15 minutes to an hour after injection and they stay active the body for three to five hours depending on which one you use. They reach a peak in their action within one and two and a half hours after injection.

Fast-acting insulin is the "magic bullet" when it comes to controlling blood sugars. Used properly, fast-acting insulin can eliminate dangerous post-meal spikes. Many people with Type 2 Diabetes will find that when they control post-meal spikes their fasting blood sugar will decrease, too. So after they add a fast-acting insulin to their regimen, they need a lot less basal insulin.

But in order to use fast-acting insulin correctly, you have to be intelligent. You have to learn, with the help of your doctor or Certified Diabetes Educator, how many grams of carbohydrate are covered by one unit of your fast-acting insulin. You have to learn how to accurately assess how many grams of carbohydrate you are eating in a meal. You have to always err on the side of caution, because if you use too much fast-acting insulin you *can* have nasty hypos.

Dr. Bernstein makes the point in his book, *Dr. Bernstein's Diabetes Solution,* that the only way to use fast-acting insulin safely is to use it with a lowered carbohydrate intake. This is because the more carbohydrate you eat, the more likely you are to be wrong when you estimate how many grams of carbohydrate are on your plate. And the more wrong you are about how much carbohydrate you are eating, the more likely you are to inject the wrong dose of insulin.

Another problem with injected insulin involves the speed with which it is absorbed from the injection site into the blood. The larger the dose, the slower it may absorb. Ideally you want the glucose from your food to hit the bloodstream at the same time as the insulin does. To make that happen, you must be aware of the absorption speed of the particular insulin you are injecting — they are all slightly different — and must know how fast the food you ate will digest.

This is why meal-time insulin is tricky. Let's say you want to eat a plate of spaghetti and sauce. You estimate that it contains 80 grams of carbohydrate. Your CDE told you that, for you, one unit of insulin should cover 5 grams of carbohydrate. So you inject 16 units of Novolog insulin. Novolog usually starts to work about 15 minutes after you eat. But because pasta digests very slowly, that insulin may arrive in the bloodstream long before the glucose from the pasta gets there. Now you have 16 units of insulin in your bloodstream but almost no glucose there. So you are likely to end up with a hypo.

Alternatively, you may inject enough Humulin R to match the 70 grams of glucose contained in a bagel, only to discover that the bagel digested so quickly that the glucose from it hit your bloodstream *before* the insulin was absorbed from the injection site. This will cause you to experience a high blood sugar spike. Then, a few hours later when all the insulin has been absorbed from that injection site, you may experience low blood sugar. This happens because like most Type 2s, you still produce a small second-phase insulin release that may kick in occasionally—and unpredictably—after you eat. If that second-phase insulin response mops up some of the glucose from the bagel before the delayed injected insulin gets to it, you'll end up with more insulin in your system than glucose, and then, once again, it's hypo time.

And this doesn't even get into the question of what happens if that plate of spaghetti you ate only contained 50 grams of carbohydrate instead of the 80 grams you dosed for.

This should make it clear why using fast-acting insulin to cover meals is tricky. It also makes it clear why smart insulin users keep their carbohydrate intake relatively low. A lower carbohydrate content requires a smaller insulin dose. And when you use a small dose of insulin, if you don't quite match the insulin to the food, the lower dose of insulin you have injected is not as likely to cause a serious hypo or leave you with a serious blood sugar spike.

This also should make it clear that it takes time to learn to use fast-acting insulin. You must learn how long it takes injected insulin to hit your bloodstream. You must learn how much insulin to use for the different foods you eat. You must learn how various medications you take can change your response to your insulin. But if you have the patience to learn how to use fast-acting insulin, you can get extremely good control. Many of us do and are very grateful for it.

Pre-Mixed Insulins

Doctors sometimes start patients out on so-called premixed insulins. They usually have the phrase "70/30" in their name. These insulins are mixtures. Thirty percent of the insulin is made up of fast-acting insulin and 70% of some from of NPH insulin. In theory this kind of insulin saves you money and makes it possible to use fewer shots. But because you cannot match the dose fast-acting component of the insulin to carbohydrate content of your meals without also modifying the dose of the longer acting NPH component—a kind of insulin which is notorious for causing unexpected lows, you are not likely to get good blood sugar control using a premixed insulin. If your doctor prescribes it, give it a try, but if you have trouble making it work, ask your doctor to prescribe separate basal and fast-acting insulins.

Regular Human Insulin and Analog Insulin

One more issue that you need to understand is the difference between the newer insulins which have come onto the market over the last decade and the older kind. The new insulins are what are called **insulin analogs.** The older insulin is called **regular human insulin**.

Analog insulins consist of genetically engineered molecules that are not identical to the insulin your body makes. These analog insulins include specially designed amino acid chains that have been added to the backbone of the original human insulin molecule. These amino acid chains, which are not found in the insulin your body makes, change the absorption characteristics of the analog insulin. They may cause it to be absorbed more quickly if it is a fast-acting insulin or slow the absorption if it is a basal insulin. Humalog, Novolog, Apidra, Lantus, and Levemir are all analog insulins. Each uses a different added amino acid chain to achieve its goal.

The insulin sold under the name, "Regular Human Insulin" or **R insulin,** contains molecules identical to the insulin your body makes. Humulin and Novolin R are brand names for the fastest form of regular human insulin. NPH insulin is a slower-acting form of regular human insulin. It has been treated with zinc and a protein called protamine to slow down its absorption. All the regular human insulins are much cheaper than analogs. Novolin R is available for about $22 a vial at Wal-Mart while Humalog or Novolog may be $60 or more per vial.

Though R insulin is a fast-acting insulin, the analog fast-acting insulins are much faster than R. Their concentration in the bloodstream may peak more sharply than does R and at less predictable times. Even so, most people who can afford them prefer analog fast-acting insulins because of their speed. Though they work best if you give them ten or fifteen minutes before you start eating, you can inject Humalog or Novolog right before you take your first bite. In contrast, if you use regular human insulin, you may have to inject 45 minutes to an hour before you eat to ensure that the insulin meets up properly with the food.

The slower analog basal insulins produce much steadier blood sugars than NPH does and they last longer, too.

But even so, there are situations in which regular human insulin may be a better choice than an analog insulin, especially if you are not eating a lot of carbohydrates. Regular human insulin is often more predictable in its action than analogs. And because it acts a bit more slowly and its concentration does not peak in the bloodstream all at once, it is less likely to cause hypos. Some people like to use an analog insulin if they are going to be eating at a restaurant and can't predict when their food will arrive, but at home, where they know exactly when they will be eating, they may prefer to use R insulin as it is a gentler in action and less likely to cause a hypo.

Regular human insulin does not get the marketing push the expensive, patented analog insulins get. So your doctor may have been convinced by drug company salespeople that it is "obsolete" and be unfamiliar with how to prescribe it. But it is far from obsolete. You can get very good control with regular human insulin.

You need a prescription to buy any analog insulin, but in most states in the U.S. you can buy regular human insulin without a prescription, though you might need a prescription for the needles you will need to inject it. Wal-mart pharmacies sell a cheap store brand version of regular human insulin which is much cheaper than the brand name insulin you buy elsewhere.

Non-Injected Forms of Insulin

Inhalable insulin was introduced to the market with great fanfare in 2005, but failed miserably, mostly because the inhalable version was supposed to be a fast-acting meal-time insulin, but it was extremely difficult to match it to the carbohydrate in a meal. It was also priced even more exorbitantly than the analog insulins. The high price and the mediocre performance kept insurers from covering it. It was subsequently taken off the market.

There are several new formulations of non-injected insulin which are undergoing various stages of testing, including some oral forms of insulin that are supposedly absorbed through the cheek tissue. Before you get too excited about any new form of fast-acting insulin, ask how long it takes to reach the bloodstream and how closely the dose can be matched to the food you eat with it. If the speed and match are good, these new insulins may be a wonderful improvement for people with diabetes, but history suggests this is a very big "if."

Treating Mild Hypos

Everyone who is using insulin should learn how to treat a mild hypo. A mild hypo occurs when you have taken slightly more insulin than you needed and your blood sugar is drifting below normal. Your doctor should tell you at what blood sugar level you should correct a mild hypo. For many of us, that level is below 75 mg/dl. There is no need to correct blood sugars in the 80s unless your blood sugar is dropping very quickly and you know your insulin will not stop working for a while longer.

If you have injected a much larger dose of insulin than you intended, or have mistakenly injected fast-acting insulin instead of your basal insulin, you could have a severe hypo. In that case, call your doctor immediately or get someone to drive you to an emergency room!

The best way to treat a hypo is to use pure glucose. It will reach your bloodstream within a few minutes. Use only enough to bring your blood sugar back to a safe level. For most of us a good target for a safe blood sugar level is no higher than 110 mg/dl.

Learn How Much Glucose Raises Your Blood Sugar 10 mg/dl

The amount of glucose that raises your blood sugar a given amount depends on your body weight. Use the table below to find the amount of glucose you will need to eat to raise your blood sugar 10 mg/dl.

Your Weight (lbs)	Glucose Needed (g)
140	2
175	2.5
210	3
245	3.5
280	4
315	4.5

Table 4. Glucose Needed to Raise Blood Sugar 10 mg/dl

How to Get Your Glucose

You can get two grams of glucose in five American "Smarties" candy discs or one hard "Sweetart" candy wafer. It is listed as "dextrose" on the label. Check the nutritional information on the wrapper to be sure it hasn't changed.

You can also buy glucose tablets at the drug store. However, the good thing about Smarties and Sweetarts is that in an emergency you can buy them at gas stations and convenience stores. If you use insulin, keep a roll in your pocket or your purse at all times.

After You've Taken the Glucose

After you've taken enough glucose to raise your blood sugar from its current level to 110 mg/dl, wait fifteen minutes and measure your blood sugar again. It should be where you wanted it to be unless whatever caused your hypo is still having an effect. If this is the case, take another dose of glucose of a size that will to move you back up to your safety blood sugar level.

Why Not Just Eat Two Grams of Any Carbohydrate-Containing Food?

It is best to use pure glucose because it is the only sugar that goes directly into your blood stream and does not require the time-consuming digestion that sucrose, lactose, fructose, or starch require. Glucose is already in the form that goes into the bloodstream.

If you try to raise your blood sugar with starchy or sugary food, the carbohydrate not only needs to be digested, it is mixed up with proteins or fats that will slow its digestion. Milk also needs digestion.

If you have been restricting your carbs very tightly, you may look upon a hypo as an opportunity to eat a high carbohydrate treat, such as a piece of cake. This is a bad habit to get into. Treat hypos with speedy glucose. If you want a piece of cake, schedule one in as an off plan indulgence.

Eating food to counter frequent mild hypos can cause weight gain. There are only four calories in a gram of glucose. So even if you take 12 grams, you are only going to get 48 calories. But if you start eating starchy and sugary food to correct frequent lows, you are likely to eat far more calories and over time those calories will add up. This may be one reason why drugs that cause hypos, like insulin and sulfonylureas are associated with weight gain.

Chapter Ten
Supplements and Healing Foods

Can Special Foods and Expensive Supplements Control Your Diabetes?

Because cutting down on carbohydrates makes such a huge difference in your blood sugars, it's easy to believe there must be other foods and supplements that would have an equally powerful effect and which might even be powerful enough to let you work that fudge sundae back into your food plan.

But such foods and supplements don't exist. What does exist is a huge industry looking to make money off you and other people with chronic diseases, an industry that profits mightily from selling you worthless remedies at highly inflated prices. Many of them advertise using Google Ads. Their products line the shelves of so-called "Health Food" stores, and articles about them fill many pages of magazines devoted to alternative healing.

If you're newly diagnosed, it's almost certain that you are going to shell out for some of their products. They promise so much, and you're only human! But before you head down to the health food store and drain your bank account, consider the following.

Why You Need to Be Suspicious of Dietary Research Boosting Specific Foods and Supplements

Though the media often report that one or another food or supplement prevents or cures diabetes, these reports are almost always based on press releases touting studies funded by the companies who sell the food or supplement. The press rarely reports on the work of independent academic researchers who call these claims into question or disprove them.

For example, you have undoubtedly read many articles suggesting that eating soy products can help women with menopausal symptoms. But you probably did not see the research that showed that those same soy products can be toxic to the thyroid glands of those same menopausal women or that eating soy products may make you more susceptible to developing food allergies. For that matter, you probably didn't see the research done by scientists not funded by the soy producers that cast doubt on whether soy really was even effective for countering menopausal symptoms.

There are virtually no investigative journalists working in the medical press. Newspapers and TV networks turn press releases into "news" without scrutinizing the studies they cite to see if they pass the most basic tests of scientific validity. When you see a doctor commenting on these press release news items, they are often doctors on the payroll of the companies who sent out the press release.

The Supplement Business is Rife with Fraud

Even if a supplement really lives up to its health claims, there is no guarantee that the product you paid for is in the capsule that you bought. In fact, it is likely that it isn't. That is because the supplement business in the United States is completely unregulated.

Back in the 1980s the United States Congress, at the behest of a powerful senator whose campaigns receive significant funding from a huge Utah supplement manufacturer, forbade the FDA from regulating supplements. The government can step in only when a supplement is so dangerous that it kills a large number of people. This was the case with the tryptophan sleep supplements which in the late 1980s killed 37 people and left 1,500 more crippled. But if a supplement isn't lethal, the FDA has no authority over its manufacturers. It can't inspect factories or require tests to make sure that supplement manufacturers are really selling you the ingredients listed on their labels, though the FDA can do this for prescription drugs. The analyses run by watchdog groups often find that bottles of supplements contain a lot less of whatever it is they are supposed to contain than what is listed on the label. Even worse, the bottle may contain other substances not listed which may be harmful to you.

Buying your supplements from a brand name company doesn't guarantee purity, either. Because there are almost no American factories left that manufacture vitamins, most supplement companies buy the vitamins and the other ingredients that go into supplements from factories in China. Like all pharmaceuticals from China, they are often manufactured in substandard facilities where products are contaminated with pesticides from the polluted water used in the manufacturing process as well as solvents and industrial chemicals.

Some Chinese factories have even been known to put cheap prescription drugs into supplements to make them appear effective. Sulfonylureas and statins are among the drugs that have been found to have been added to "herbal" preparations intended to lower blood sugar or control cholesterol.

Another major problem with herbal supplements is that while they may be "natural" that doesn't mean they don't contain substances that might be bad for you. For example, there are several Chinese herbs that are effective in lowering blood sugar. They do this because they contain naturally occurring sulfonylurea molecules. So they also stimulate receptors on your heart in the same way that first generation sulfonylurea drugs did—a way that increases your likelihood of having a heart attack.

Red rice yeast lowers cholesterol because it contains a natural statin. It can also cause all the nasty side effects of a prescription statin. The only difference between taking these "natural" supplements and the prescription drugs they mimic is that when you take the supplement version you can't know what dose you are getting. The lack of regulation means that the dose of the effective component in the supplement may vary from pill to pill.

With these warnings in mind, lets look at some of the foods and supplements that are touted as helping you control your blood sugar. We will start with the most popular—and least effective.

Cinnamon

The idea that cinnamon might have some effect on blood sugar was first demonstrated in the lab by researchers at the Human Nutrition Research Center of the FDA in Beltsville Maryland in 1990. They were testing foods for an insulin-enhancing effect as part of a series of studies. Cinnamon was only one of several foods they described as having an insulin-enhancing effect. Others included peanut butter and tuna fish. The article reporting these results was published in an obscure journal and attracted no media attention.

Dr. Richard A. Anderson, a researcher connected with the USDA, then conducted a series of experiments with cinnamon which appeared to show that it could have a significant impact on lowering blood sugar. Some graduate students working under his guidance performed a study in Peshawar Pakistan which supposedly proved that two doses a day of ground cinnamon of the same type that you can purchase in any grocery store could make a dramatic difference in blood sugar.

However, it is worth noting that the same Dr. Anderson who conducted most of the research into the usefulness of cinnamon also has a patent on the compound found to be the active ingredient in cinnamon. His research therefore was not impartial.

As Dr. Ronald Tamler, an endocrinologist and editor of the PRESENT Diabetes Web newsletter, pointed out in an editorial, Dr. Anderson's very small studies that found a favorable effect from cinnamon only measured *fasting blood sugar*. Dr. Tamler cites a more recent study, whose title says it all: "Cinnamon supplementation does not improve glycemic control in postmenopausal Type 2 Diabetes patients." That study included glucose tolerance test results in its assessment of the efficacy of cinnamon.

Another study not performed by someone with a financial stake in cinnamon found that cinnamon doesn't even improve fasting blood sugars. Nor did it have any effect on A1c or lipids. A third study performed by researchers at the University of Oklahoma randomly assigned people with Type 2 Diabetes to take either cinnamon capsules or a placebo every day for three months. The cinnamon group took two capsules a day, each of which contained 500 milligrams of the spice. The placebo group took capsules containing wheat flour. The results of this study showed that there were no differences in the groups' average levels of blood sugar, insulin, or cholesterol.

Cinnamon appears to be an over-hyped underperforming supplement. But at least it has the advantage that it is one you can test at home safely and cheaply since Dr. Anderson's research, no matter how questionable, was done with plain cinnamon of the type you buy at the grocery store. Keep your dose to one teaspoon a day or less, and if you have high blood pressure be sure to monitor it. Contrary to Dr. Anderson's claims that cinnamon lowers blood pressure, some people who have tested it have reported seeing their blood pressure go up after taking cinnamon. Do not use cinnamon if you have any issues related to bleeding, as cinnamon contains a substance related to coumarin, a blood thinner.

Don't bother with the $30 bottles of cinnamon extract sold by supplement companies. They may claim that their products contain exotic forms of cinnamon that differ from what you can buy at the grocery store. But Dr. Anderson has stated in interviews that the stuff you buy at the grocery store is what he and his students used in the original research that found benefits in cinnamon.

Chromium

There was a flurry of excitement about chromium in the 1990s, after the same Dr. Anderson who got such impressive results with cinnamon reported that chromium supplementation could significantly improve glucose tolerance.

Studies conducted by Dr. Anderson and other researchers around the world seemed to show that adding chromium to the diets of people with diabetes in India and China lowered their blood sugar significantly. However, other studies with European and American populations did not show chromium having any such effect.

In his review of the chromium studies published in the *Journal of the American College of Nutrition*, published in 1998, Anderson argued that to be effective chromium should be given in the form of chromium picolinate rather than less active chromium chloride and that the minimum dose must be at least 400 micrograms and possibly as much as 1,000 mc. This dose, he said could reduce insulin resistance in people with impaired glucose tolerance and lower the blood sugar of people with Type 2 Diabetes. Anderson explained that the mechanism behind this improvement was that chromium supplementation increases the number of insulin receptors in cells.

However, despite Anderson's enthusiasm for chromium—his name was on many of the relevant research papers—none of these studies were particularly impressive. All were small. None of them involved more than 85 people and few involved more than 30.

The media—probably responding to press releases from supplement manufacturers—picked up on this and other research in 1998 and publicized it in a way that suggested that chromium supplementation not only would reduce insulin resistance but that it would also improve the speed with which dieters lost weight. Sales of chromium picolinate skyrocketed.

But few dieters found the supplement to be all that effective, and a subsequent review of the research by NIH statisticians, M.D. Althuis and N.E. Jordan concluded that chromium supplementation had no effect on glucose or insulin levels in non-diabetic people and that the evidence for an effect on people with diabetes was inconclusive.

Some researchers speculated that the results seen in the Chinese and

Indian studies might have been due to these particular populations subsisting on mediocre diets that were deficient in chromium. The diet eaten by most people in the First World supplies more than enough chromium.

Chromium's role as a supplement was dealt a death blow by the discovery that chromium picolinate caused mutations of a type that leads to cancer in hamsters and fruit flies. More recent research has called this result into question and the current belief is that small amounts of chromium picolinate are probably safe, though not likely to do much for you unless you are chromium deficient.

If you want to test chromium you can buy inexpensive chromium picolinate at the drug store. Try one package and if you don't see a significant change, you'll know it isn't worth investing in.

Even better, the safest approach to chromium supplementation—as is the case with most mineral supplementation—is to get chromium through the foods you eat. Foods rich in chromium that won't raise your blood sugar include seafood, green beans, broccoli, nuts, and peanut butter, all of which contain other helpful micronutrients. Eating foods that contain vitamin C, like berries or green pepper, may increase the absorption of dietary chromium.

If a supplement company claims you can't get the health benefits of some nutrient by eating several servings a day of foods that contain it, be skeptical. Over and over again research comes up with the finding that nutrients originally identified as having health benefits when they were taken in the form of food are worthless when taken in pills.

For example, people eating a lot of vegetables containing beta carotene appeared to suffer less lung cancer than those who did not. But when the beta carotene was administered in the form of vitamin pills no such effect was demonstrated. There are many micronutrients in any real food which are not included in pills and it is possible they work together synergistically.

Antioxidants

Many small scale studies have shown that the antioxidant vitamins C and E may have some effect in preventing heart disease. However, a large scale study conducted in England where half of 20,536 people considered high risk for heart disease took vitamin C, E, and beta-carotene supplements and half didn't, has cast a great deal of doubt on this.

Despite the fact that those in the supplemented group had measurably higher blood levels of the supplemented vitamins, the researchers found no difference at all in their rates of heart attack, other signs of cardiovascular disease, cancer or, indeed, hospitalization for any other cause.

A separate study published in February of 2007, in contrast, found that antioxidant supplements actually seemed to *raise* the risk of death in those who took them. The reasons for this are unknown, but since Vitamin C and most other vitamins are no longer produced by factories located in the United States but are instead manufactured in China, it is quite possible that toxic contaminants like pesticides or industrial chemicals that made their way into the vitamin pills used in these studies caused the higher rates of death.

There is still some evidence that supplementing with these vitamins might be of some use to people with diabetes. Studies have certainly shown that the beta cell is uniquely vulnerable to oxidative stress because it is poor in the production of antioxidant substances. So it has seemed reasonable to think that raising the bloodstream concentrations of these antioxidants might help counter this.

A paper published in 2000 that analyzed results of the EPIC-Norfolk Study at first suggested this was true. It found that the higher the plasma vitamin C level in the 6,458 people they studied—people both with and without diabetes—the lower their A1c seemed to be. But a further analysis of EPIC-Norfolk data published in 2004—after the results were in showing the ineffectiveness of vitamin supplementation against heart disease—made it clear that high levels of Vitamin C were markers for a healthier way of eating rather than the cause of better blood sugars.

The study title says it all: "Occupational social class, educational level and area deprivation independently predict plasma ascorbic acid concentration." In short, the better off and the better educated you are the more likely you are to eat a diet that is filled with the fruits and vegetables that raise the levels of vitamin C in your blood rather than starchy sugary junk food that raises your blood sugar.

Vitamin E Appears Effective in the Presence of a Certain Gene

One reason for the confusing results described above in large-scale studies of antioxidants became clear in November of 2007. A team in Israel discovered that people with one particular gene, the haptoglobin

(Hp) 2-2 gene, who took 400 iu of Vitamin E, had 40% less heart attacks over an 18 month period than those who did not have that particular gene.

So if you are going to supplement these vitamins, use low doses. Dr. Bernstein warns against taking doses of vitamin C greater than 500 mg a day, explaining that very high levels of vitamin C can raise blood sugar and impair nerve function. He writes that vitamin E in doses between 400 to 1,200 IU per day may lower insulin resistance, but suggests you use gamma tocopherol or mixed tocopherols, not the commonly found version of Vitamin E, alpha tocopherol, which he says can inhibit the absorption of gamma tocopherol from food.

Get Your Antioxidants from Food

Because of the problems with vitamin manufacturers and because your body evolved over millions of years during which nutrients did not arrive in pill form, you are much more likely to get whatever health benefits there are in any nutrient if you get that nutrient from the foods it occurs in naturally.

To get antioxidants from food, consume nuts and sunflower seeds which are an excellent source of vitamin E. You can get adequate amounts of vitamin C from green vegetables, small servings of tomato, and low carbohydrate fruits like blueberries, raspberries, and strawberries.

Magnesium

An analysis of data from the Nurses Health Study suggests that increased intake of dietary magnesium corresponded with a reduced risk of diabetes. This result was echoed by a similar finding analyzing data from another study, the Iowa Women's Health Study. Adequate blood levels of magnesium have also been found to counter high blood pressure.

However, again it is not clear whether high blood magnesium levels truly prevent blood sugar deterioration or are simply a marker that a person does not have the underlying conditions that cause abnormal blood sugars.

A new concern about supplementing minerals, including magnesium, is the finding published in January of 2008 that calcium supplementation at the high levels currently recommended appears to increase the incidence of heart attacks in older women. This may be because excess calcium gets deposited as hard plaque in the arteries.

Since blood magnesium levels affect calcium levels, it may be a mistake to supplement either of these minerals with pills. Get your magnesium from the nuts and leafy green vegetables you should be eating for all the other good things they contain. Plentiful amounts of magnesium are also found in premium chocolates with high cocoa content.

Fructose

You may be told by ignorant nutritionists that fructose is preferable to other sugars for people with diabetes because it doesn't raise insulin or blood sugar. Fructose is a simple sugar which is found in fruits, and for this reason it has been promoted as being "natural" and "healthy." However the fructose you find listed in the ingredient panel of supermarket foods does not come from fruit. It is extracted from corn. And no matter what the source of fructose, it turns out that no form of fructose is good for people with diabetes.

This is because while it is true that fructose may not raise your blood glucose concentration, upon being digested fructose makes a beeline for the liver where it is immediately turned into fat. Not only that, but dietary fructose also increases insulin resistance and decreases leptin, a hormone that regulates appetite and body fat levels.

The reason humans are so drawn to fructose probably goes back to our evolutionary primate heritage. Fat is hard to come by for most primates as they don't eat much meat. And stored body fat may be what gets that primate through times when food is scarce. Primates get a lot of their body fat from the fructose in the fruits they consume and they are very motivated to find fruit, possibly because of how badly they need that fat.

But when our bodies start encountering "fruit" sugar in large quantities every day though we never run into times when food is scarce, this becomes a problem. Our brains certainly seem to be hardwired to eat as much fructose as possible. Table sugar is one half fructose one half glucose, which may explain why it is so seductively attractive.

The average consumption of fructose by Americans rose from 64 grams per day in 1970 to 81 grams per day in 1997—a rise of 26%—and that was just the *average* consumption. Anyone who starts their day with glass of orange juice and cereal sweetened with high fructose corn syrup, and then drinks a soda with lunch, eats a dinner that includes canned soup or bottled spaghetti sauce—all of which are sweetened with surprising amounts of high fructose corn syrup—and then polishes off that meal with a scoop of ice cream or cookies which are also sweetened with high fructose corn syrup is taking in a lot more fructose than that 81 gram average.

There is an accumulating body of research which suggests that because fructose may deregulate the built in controls on appetite and because it causes increased fat storage, the huge increase in fructose consumption over the past couple decades may have a lot to do with the concomitant increase in obesity within the U.S population. You can read a lot more about what researchers have found about the effects of fructose on your body in Gary Taubes' book, *Good Calories, Bad Calories.*

Selenium May Raise Diabetes Risk

Selenium is a mineral which had been found in some small experiments to appear to lower blood sugar. However, a study published in July of 2007, which attempted to see whether long term supplementation with selenium would prevent Type 2 Diabetes, discovered that it appeared to do just the opposite. The group taking the selenium supplements developed more diabetes. Not only that, but the more selenium in their blood plasma, the more likely people were to develop diabetes. Strike selenium off your list of supplements for diabetes, unless you want to *get* diabetes.

Herbs

Herbs you'll see routinely touted as helping diabetes include the herb Gymnema Sylvestre and the Indian spice, Fenugreek. You can try sprinkling fenugreek on your food to see if it helps you. It is sold as a spice and it can be found in fresh form at Indian grocery stores. The fresh leaves are preferable, as they are eaten as a normal part of diets in some parts of the world and anecdotal evidence is that the leaves may lower blood sugar.

But here, as in the case of most herbs, there is always the possibility that these herbs lower blood sugar in ways that are not good for you, for example, by over-stimulating the beta cells. As noted diabetes author Gretchen Becker has pointed out, many "natural" cures popular in India work because they damage the liver. When the liver is damaged it no longer dumps glucose into your bloodstream, so your blood sugar drops. Unfortunately, as the damage continues, your liver no longer removes toxins from your blood and barring a liver transplant, you die.

Vanadyl Sulfate is another supplement that has been found to lower blood sugar but does it by damaging the body.

The supplements we are about to discuss next are those where either peer-reviewed research or strong anecdotal reports suggest that they may have some benefit for people with diabetes.

Benfotiamine

Benfotiamine is a supplement for which there is a growing amount of research suggesting that it might be helpful for people with diabetes. In particular it appears to help neuropathic pain and may reduce the incidence of microvascular complications.

Benfotiamine is a lipid soluble form of thiamine or vitamin B-1. One study has found that the blood of people with diabetes is very deficient in vitamin B-1 (thiamine) and explained that this had been missed in previous testing for technical reasons. Other research suggests that thiamine can block the processes that lead to the microvascular complications, neuropathy, retinopathy, and kidney disease.

Recommended Dose:

The dose used in the experiments with humans that found benefits in benfotiamine varies. In one such study the dose was "two 50 mg benfotiamine tablets four times daily" (400 mg/day). In another it was "a combination of benfotiamine (100 mg) and pyridoxine hydrochloride (100 mg)" once a day.

Alpha Lipoic Acid

This expensive supplement has been used in intravenous form to treat neuropathy in Germany. It is an insulin mimic—i.e. it appears to stimulate some of the same receptors insulin does. It is also an antioxidant. In a German study, doctors from Buhl and City Hospital in Baden-Baden administered different dosages of oral ALA and placebo to 74 patients for four weeks. They then tested their insulin levels and found that the ability to take up glucose improved by an average of 27% in the people taking the ALA compared to the placebo group. All the dosages they tested appeared equally effective. The lowest dose used was 600 mg taken once a day. However, this is still a very small study, and a published review of other studies found less conclusive results for ALA taken orally rather than intravenously.

Dr. Bernstein writes that he has his patients take ALA in combination with Evening Primrose Oil to potentiate the action of insulin whether it is the insulin produced by their own bodies or injected.

When I have scanned the Web for discussions about this supplement I have not turned up much encouraging news about its effect on enhancing insulin sensitivity. Many people report that the combination of ALA and EPO caused them intolerable gastric distress, EPO was reported to cause mood swings by others, and almost no one reports seeing significant changes in blood sugar after taking this expensive supplement pair.

Some people with Type 2 Diabetes do report that ALA helps them with neuropathic pain and that it does not seem to matter whether they use the time release or regular form. There is an isomer of ALA, R-ALA which is supposed to be more bio-available. Dr. Bernstein recommends using this form, which is marketed in the U.S. under the brand name, "Insulow." Several people have posted enthusiastically about it.

One Caution About ALA

An editorial in the Japanese Journal 'Internal Medicine'" warns that in people with a specific genetic makeup that makes them extremely likely to develop autoimmune (Type 1) diabetes, ALA may provoke an antibody attack. The explanation for why this happens is that "a-lipoic acid (ALA) is reduced in the body to a sulfhydryl compound" and that sulfur rich compounds stimulate the immune attack. This does not appear to be a concern for people who do not have a strong history of autoimmune diabetes.

Recommended Dose:

The Baden-Baden study cited above used 600 mg orally once a day. *Dr. Bernstein's Diabetes Solution* currently recommends two 100 mg tablets every 8 hours to be taken along with one 500 mg capsule of Evening Primrose oil.

Foods that Heal?

After your diabetes diagnosis, you'll be much more likely to notice the never-ending stream of reports in the media about how this or that food has healing properties. Can you really use dark chocolate to control your blood pressure and yogurt to keep your blood sugar in line?

Alas, the answer in every case is "No, not if you actually want to make significant improvements."

Even worse, the research on which manufacturers base their claims is often seriously flawed and intentionally misleading. So eating the foods they promote as being good for diabetes may actually worsen your condition.

A Perfect Example of a Perfectly Flawed Study: "Soy Yogurt Could Help Control Diabetes"

This news item, which was distributed by the AP in November of 2006, is a good example of how industry uses poorly conducted research to support specious health claims for questionable products. It was titled, "Soy Yogurt Could Help Control Diabetes" and its conclusion was that blueberry soy yogurt "controls diabetes" because it contains more of a specific phytochemical that inhibits the enzymes that break down sugar than do the other fruit yogurts it was compared to.

What's striking here is that the researchers drew their conclusion that their yogurt "controlled diabetes" by measuring the amount of this phytochemical in the yogurts. They did not observe the effect of any of the sugary fruit-filled yogurts on anyone's blood sugar. Since both regular and soy fruit yogurt are full of sugar—usually 23 grams per serving, any yogurt will raise blood sugar way beyond the ability of any phytochemical to lower it.

The researchers who performed this study also claimed that their soy blueberry yogurt lowered ACE, a hormone involved in the regulation of blood pressure, more than did other sugary yogurts. Perhaps it also lowered ACE levels a few micrograms more than did Milky Ways and chocolate cake. This does *not* make it a drug in food form. But based only on the tiny effect they observed their yogurt to have on ACE, the company also claimed that their sugary fruit yogurt lowered blood pressure. This conclusion was not arrived at by measuring blood pressure in any human beings who had eaten their yogurt.

The study did not mention that soy can be toxic to marginal thyroid glands and that people with Type 2 Diabetes have a high incidence of thyroid disease and should therefore avoid eating soy foods.

The medical press publishes these kinds of studies without subjecting them to any kind of critical analysis. The company press release is printed word for word as if it were a news story. By the time the story reaches the TV audience it has been stripped of any facts you could use to assess its validity.

Does Dark Chocolate Control Blood Pressure?

If you have diabetes, controlling your blood pressure is the next most important thing you can do to keep yourself healthy after controlling your blood sugar. So you probably were thrilled on July 4, 2007, when you saw some version of this headline in your newspaper: "Dark Chocolate lowers blood pressure!" But before you hit the Hershey's, it's worth taking a look at those pesky details.

In this study, test participants were divided into two groups. One consumed a daily dose of dark chocolate; the other the same amount of white chocolate. Then every day for 18 weeks, the volunteers were instructed to eat one-square portions of a 16-square Ritter Sport bar, or a similar portion of white chocolate, which doesn't contain cocoa. Note the way the brand name was featured prominently in this "news" story.

After consuming their square of Ritter Sport dark chocolate every day, the subjects' average systolic blood pressure fell nearly three points and their average diastolic blood pressure dropped almost two points This isn't much of an improvement, but still, it is something. But here's the kicker. The subjects' *average* blood pressure at the start of the 18-week test was *147/ 86*. This means that at the end of the study the average blood pressure of those eating the chocolate had been lowered only to 144 /82, which as any doctor will confirm is still too high!

So here's what the journalists who reported this study should have been asking: Why were people with damagingly high blood pressures allowed to maintain those damagingly high blood pressures for 18 weeks instead of being put on one of the many effective drugs that would have lowered their blood pressure? What were the ethics of the doctors who subjected these patients to such a study?

I like chocolate as much as the next woman, possibly more. So, trust me, if dark chocolate had healing properties, I'd be healed! But all this study really proved is that eating chocolate is not an effective way to get better blood pressure control. And when the chocolate companies are rolling out $3 chocolate bars plastered with health claims, this is worth keeping in mind.

"Healthy" Whole Grains

There are hundreds of other examples of the way this kind of manipulative "science" has been put into the service of selling you question-able products posing as healing foods. The most dangerous for people with diabetes are those used to promote so called "healthy whole grains."

There are many studies purporting to prove that whole grains have enormous health benefits, especially for people with diabetes. In all these studies the researchers compare the effects of eating a whole grain food with those of eating a highly processed food with even more carbohydrate per serving than is found in the whole grain.

So yes, a study may prove that whole grain toast is slightly easier on your blood sugar than Sugar Frosted Flakes. But if you were to compare a breakfast made up of whole grain toast and oatmeal to one containing scrambled eggs and ham, the real effect of those "healthy" whole gains on your health would quickly become apparent. Anyone with a blood sugar meter can quickly establish whether or not any supposedly healing food is healthy. If it raises your blood sugar over your blood sugar target, it isn't.

Chapter Eleven
Exercise

Every book, every article, and every doctor will tell you that you should control your diabetes with "diet and exercise," and it is quite true that exercise is a valuable tool for controlling your blood sugar. Exercise may increase the insulin sensitivity of your muscles both while you exercise and for a few hours afterwards. It also builds more muscle, and having more muscle will help you burn off more glucose and may increase your insulin sensitivity overall.

Most people think that "exercise" means going to the gym, and indeed, for many people, the weight training and endurance aerobics you can do with the help of the machines you find at a gym may be helpful. But if you have had high blood sugars for a while and have long been sedentary, an aggressive program of gym exercise may end up giving you serious injuries that make future exercise almost impossible.

Gym exercises can also raise your heart rate dramatically, which can pose a problem if you do not start out very gradually and improve your cardiovascular fitness in small steps. Be sure to get your doctor's approval before you start a new exercise regimen. If you use machines that can measure heart rate, keep an eye on your heart rate and make sure it is not higher than the 50 to 75% of the maximum heart rate that is safe for a person of your age. The American Heart Association states that a healthy person's maximum heart rate should be 220 minus their age. If you have been diagnosed with heart disease your doctor must tell you what heart rate is safe for you.

The Best Exercise is Exercise that Avoids Injury

People with diabetes or prediabetes who have experienced years of undiagnosed high blood sugars are very prone to develop tendon problems. This may be because high blood sugars cause tendons to become brittle. There is also some evidence that years of exposure to even slightly elevated blood sugars cause abnormal thickening of tendons.

Some of the tendon problems that are very common among people with diabetes are frozen shoulder, carpal tunnel syndrome, tarsal tunnel syndrome, and piriformis syndrome. These are what doctors call "entrapment syndromes." Thickened tendons compress nerves that pass through narrow openings which causes pain or numbness. Some of these syndromes, like frozen shoulder,* may resolve over time, but carpal tunnel syndrome can result in permanent nerve damage.

Piriformis syndrome is an entrapment syndrome where a nerve that passes down the hip into the leg gets compressed and causes sciatic pain. Dr. Loren Fishman, a researcher who authored the book, *Sciatica Solutions*, claims that piriformis syndrome is often the source of back pain that is misdiagnosed as being caused by vertebral disc problems. Dr. Richard K. Bernstein has written an essay stating that piriformis syndrome is especially common among people with diabetes. Though vertebral discs that rupture are surprisingly rare, Dr. Fishman also writes that when these discs do rupture it may be a result of high blood sugar weakening the material making up the vertebral discs.

If you are an older person with diabetes who may have had undiagnosed high blood sugars for many years, you are likely to have fragile tendons throughout your body and should be very careful to avoid exercise that puts abnormal stress on your tendons and joints. Walking is better than running, because it is much less likely to damage your knees. If you walk, walk briskly on paths or sidewalks, if possible, rather than on the hard, artificial surface of the treadmill. Too much treadmilling may cause repetitive stress damage in your feet.

If you lift weights, don't be overly zealous. Do enough to increase your fitness but avoid damaging those vulnerable shoulders, vertebral discs, and knees. Don't trust that the muscular young "instructors" at your gym know what they are talking about. Many have only a very limited education in exercise physiology and may know nothing about the problems of exercising with fragile tendons or an iffy back.

Study after study shows that half an hour of brisk walking five times a week will give you all the physiological benefits of exercise without damaging your joints.

---

* Though many doctors don't know this, both frozen shoulder and carpal tunnel syndrome may be the first symptom of abnormal blood sugars. One study found that a diagnosis of carpel tunnel syndrome typically occurred ten years before a formal diagnosis of diabetes. If you get a frozen shoulder resist the temptation to treat it surgically. Frozen shoulder usually resolves on its own over a period lasting six months to a year. There is no evidence that painful physical therapy regimens speed up the natural healing process.

10,000 Steps

Some people with diabetes have found it very helpful to snap a pedometer on their belt and use it to count their steps. The goal is to gradually increase the number of steps you take each day until you have gotten up to 10,000 steps a day.

That amount of walking is enough to provide health benefits, especially if you can keep it up month in and month out. Wearing the pedometer will encourage you to walk in situations where you might otherwise ride, to park farther from the office or store, and to take a few turns around the mall when it is rainy and there is nothing else to do.

Swimming is another very healthy exercise that many people find they can do without injuring their joints.

When You Can't Exercise

If, like many older people, you have orthopedic problems that make it extremely difficult to exercise, you may become depressed by the thought that your lack of mobility means you won't be able to lose weight or get good control of your diabetes.

This turns out not to be true.

I managed to lose 18% of my starting body weight without doing any exercise and I was able to maintain that loss for almost five years. Exercise has many benefits, but it is nowhere near as helpful in attaining weight loss as people selling gym memberships would have you believe.

A book that followed successful dieters who had lost a lot of weight and kept it off more than five years found that few of the successful women dieters did any exercise until they reached their weight goals though many of them used exercise to help them maintain their weight loss over time.

Not only can you lose weight with out exercise, but it is also possible to reach your blood sugar goals without it, though exercise is a great tool for burning off unexpected blood sugars highs.

So if your mobility is limited, don't panic. Do what you can. Walk, roll, or wiggle what you can wiggle. And be really good about sticking to your diet!

Exercise and Blood Sugar Level

If you exercise energetically there are two things you need to know about how exercise affects blood sugar.

If you start exercising when your blood sugar is very high, you may end up pushing your blood sugar up even higher, rather than lowering it. This is particularly true if you are insulin deficient rather than insulin resistant. Some authorities suggest that you should not begin an exercise session when your blood sugar is over 200 mg/dl for this reason.

Use your meter to find out the impact of exercise on your own blood sugar. Test before you start your exercise session. Then check your blood sugar after every fifteen minutes of exercising. Check again when you finish and two hours later. If you see your blood sugar going up rather than down, you will know you need to lower your blood sugar before you start exercising. If you see it drop, you now have a helpful technique for correcting spikes caused by unwise eating.

If you start exercising aggressively when your blood sugar is at a normal level, you may end up with the symptoms of low blood sugar. This is a concern mainly when you are using insulin or a drug that makes the beta cells secrete insulin. Be sure to test any time you feel like you might be going low and bring some glucose tabs, Sweetarts, or Smarties with you when you exercise. Review the information on Page 136 about how to treat a mild hypo.

Avoid the temptation to correct mild hypos you experience while exercising with sugary sports drinks or juice. These contain so much sugar they may push your blood sugar up far too high. If your blood sugar goes way down and then way up while you exercise, you will end up making yourself more insulin resistant as well as ravenously hungry. You may also end up feeling drained and exhausted after an exercise session rather than refreshed.

As was the case with the diabetes diet, the diabetes exercise program should be one you can stick with for decades, long past the point where your initial enthusiasm wanes. As was the case with diet, you are most likely to succeed at exercise long term if you treat yourself gently and don't force yourself to do things you hate doing.

Find activities that improve fitness which you enjoy, and when they get boring find new ones. A steady program that increases your fitness in a modest way year in and year out is much better for a person with diabetes than indulging in a few months of aggressive over-exercising, burning out, injuring yourself, and going back to being sedentary!

Chapter Twelve
Is it Really Type 2?

If you've been diagnosed with Type 2 Diabetes but are not overweight and lack other markers of insulin resistance such as an apple-shaped distribution of body fat or a strong response to Metformin, it is possible that you don't really have Type 2 Diabetes. This is especially likely if you cut way back on your carbohydrates but still find that you are getting high post-meal blood sugars. If you have relatives who are also thin but have been diagnosed with either Type 2 or Type 1 Diabetes, this is even more likely.

There are two other forms of diabetes that are often misdiagnosed as Type 2 Diabetes. Many family doctors have not been trained to recognize them and may not even know they exist.

LADA

Latent Autoimmune Diabetes of Adults (LADA) is a slow-developing form of autoimmune diabetes that usually occurs in people over 30 years old. It is often misdiagnosed as Type 2.

Because LADA is an autoimmune form of diabetes, over time it is likely to progress to full fledged Type 1 Diabetes — the form of diabetes in which the beta cells are killed by an autoimmune attack. If there is a chance you might have LADA it is important to get the tests that could diagnose it or rule it out, since people with autoimmune diabetes can experience a life-threatening condition caused by extremely high blood sugars **called Diabetic Ketoacidosis** (DKA).[*]

Treatment for LADA is quite different from treatment for Type 2 Diabetes. It is important to start insulin treatment as early as possible if you have LADA, as there is some evidence that early insulin supplementation may lessen the immune system attack on the beta cells,

---

[*] **Diabetic ketoacidosis** (DKA) is unrelated to the "ketosis" which occurs when you are eating a very low carbohydrate diet. When you are eating a low carbohydrate diet you may have ketones in your blood and urine but your blood sugar is normal. Diabetic ketoacidosis occurs when blood sugar is extremely high. It is caused by low or nonexistant insulin levels. If you ever see a blood sugar higher than 300 mg/dl that does not drop in a few hours or continues to rise, contact your doctor immediately or go to the emergency room. DKA can be fatal. If you experience DKA it is very likely you have Type 1 Diabetes or LADA rather than Type 2 Diabetes.

which may help them survive longer. Though people with LADA must use insulin, it is much easier to use insulin when you have some residual beta cell capacity left.

Because several of the oral drugs used to treat Type 2 Diabetes stimulate the beta cells to produce insulin and because LADA involves an autoimmune attack which is worsened when the beta cells produce insulin, stimulating insulin production by the beta cells with these drugs may increase the ferocity of the attack.

So if there is any chance that you may have LADA, you should insist that your doctor run the appropriate tests and if possible refer you to an endocrinologist who is familiar with the condition.

Indicators that You May have LADA

- ❖ **A family history of Type 1 Diabetes.** There is a genetic tendency towards developing autoimmune diabetes, so if you have a close family member who has autoimmune diabetes, it is more likely that you have that same genetic makeup and the same tendency towards developing autoimmune diabetes.

- ❖ **The Presence of Other Autoimmune Conditions.** If you already have another autoimmune condition like Rheumatoid Arthritis or Autoimmune Thyroid Disease it is more likely that your diabetes is also caused by an autoimmune attack.

- ❖ **Normal or near normal weight coupled with very high blood sugars.** Although people of normal weight do develop Type 2 Diabetes many thin people in their 30s or 40s who are initially told they have Type 2 Diabetes turn out to have LADA. So LADA should always be ruled out in a thin or normal weight person diagnosed in "Type 2," especially if blood sugars are extremely high at the time of diagnosis or if blood sugars deteriorate rapidly. LADA is usually not a concern for normal weight people diagnosed with "prediabetes" unless they have a family history of Type 1 diabetes or other autoimmune conditions.

- ❖ **Failure to Respond to Oral Drugs.** People with LADA often see swift deterioration in their blood sugars in the months after a Type 2 misdiagnosis. If your blood sugars are getting worse, not better, despite taking oral drugs and cutting back on carbohydrates—the combination of treatments which is usually effective in Type 2 Diabetes, you should demand that your doctor test you for LADA or send you to an Endocrinologist who will do this.

Diagnosing LADA

The most common test for LADA is one that looks for **GAD antibodies**. GAD stands for "glutamic acid decarboxylase." A small number of people with autoimmune diabetes will not have GAD antibodies but they will have **islet cell antibodies** and/or **tyrosine phosphatase antibodies**. So a lack of GAD antibodies does not entirely rule out LADA.

The other important test for LADA is the fasting **C-peptide test**. This is a test that measures the amount of a molecule that is a byproduct of the process by which your body manufactures insulin.* A very low C-peptide result suggests that the beta cells have stopped making insulin, possibly because they are dead. People who have Type 2 Diabetes usually have test results showing normal or even high levels of C-peptide for quite a few years after their original diagnosis. So a low C-peptide level, when it occurs along with the other symptoms described above, is suggestive of LADA, though it should be confirmed with antibody tests.

Treatment for LADA

If you have LADA, the faster you get onto an insulin regimen, the better off you will be, because there's some evidence that injecting insulin will shut down your own insulin production, which in turn will keep the antibodies from attacking your beta cells and killing them off. The more beta cells you preserve, the more likely you are to benefit from future developments in treating autoimmune diabetes and possibly getting back the use of your beta cells.

If you have LADA you'd do best to get treated by an endocrinologist who specializes in treating Type 1 Diabetes, as you will need an up-to-date insulin regimen and the kind of intensive diabetes education given to people with Type 1 Diabetes.

---

* If you are not injecting insulin, a test that examines your fasting insulin level can also be helpful. People who inject insulin must take a C-peptide test as injected insulin does not contain C-peptide, so the test measures only how much insulin your body is making on its own.

MODY

A different kind of diabetes which can be mistaken for either Type 2 or Type 1 Diabetes is **Maturity Onset Diabetes of the Young** usually referred to as **MODY**. This term actually refers to several different forms of diabetes that have in common that they are genetic in origin and that they are **monogenic**. This means a person needs to inherit only a single defective gene to develop the disorder.

The defective genes that cause these various forms of MODY cause the beta cells to fail to secrete insulin. It is believed that some form of MODY may affect up to 5% of all people diagnosed with both Type 1 and Type 2 Diabetes.

Recent Research Has Changed Our Understanding of MODY

Until very recently, MODY was thought only to affect people under age 25. However, more recent genetic studies where the family members of people diagnosed with MODY were given genetic testing, turned up the fact that MODY can develop into full-fledged diabetes as late as age 55. In addition, these studies found that quite a few people carrying MODY genes had been misdiagnosed as having Type 1 or Type 2 Diabetes, depending on the age of onset and severity of their case.

A study of the age of onset of MODY-3, a more common form of MODY, found that 65% of those diagnosed were diagnosed by age 25 and 100% by age 50. So more than one third of all people with this kind of diabetes do not have symptoms severe enough to lead to a diagnosis in their youth.

Because MODY is monogenic, doctors will usually rule it out if you don't have one parent diagnosed with diabetes. But recent research has also discovered that people carrying MODY genes sometimes have blood sugar problems so mild that they escape diagnosis. So while it is true that a person with MODY usually inherits the gene from a parent who carries the MODY gene, the fact that your parent was *not* diagnosed with diabetes does not rule out the possibility that you have it, especially if other people in your family have been diagnosed with either a milder form of Type 1 Diabetes, with Type 2 Diabetes that came on when they were at a normal or near normal weight, or even with impaired glucose tolerance.

MODY genes may express less strongly if you inherited the gene from your father. That is because if the MODY gene comes from your mother she will have had gestational diabetes during the pregnancy and exposure to high blood sugars during pregnancy makes the gene express more strongly in her offspring.

How Do You Get Diagnosed with MODY?

Unfortunately, the only way to get a definitive diagnosis it to take a series of up to six very expensive genetic tests. These tests may be inconclusive since MODY experts believe there are still quite a few MODY genes other than those that current six gene tests identify. The Joslin Diabetes Center Web site states that one third of the families with the symptoms of MODY diabetes that they are following do not have one of the six genes already identified.

Many health insurers will not pay for these genetic tests, so if you cannot get MODY testing, you may have to approach a diagnosis by looking at your family history, your personal history, your weight history, and indications of how insulin resistant you are. Here are some things that might suggest there is some possibility you have MODY:

❖ If you develop diabetes though you have always been of a normal or near normal weight and tests show you have a normal fasting C-peptide level and no markers of autoimmune disease.

❖ If you have a history of gestational diabetes that occurred when you were at a normal weight.

❖ If you have close relatives who had adult onset diabetes who were of normal weight.

❖ If taking drugs that improve insulin resistance like Metformin or Actos don't make any difference in your blood sugar or A1c.

❖ If you have glucose in your urine when your blood sugar has not risen higher than 160 mg/dl after a meal, especially if there is a history of kidney disease in your family. People with MODY-3 often have subtle or even serious kidney malformations which cause them to spill glucose in their urine at relatively low blood sugars.

❖ If you have a very strong response to a sulfonylurea drug like Amaryl or Glipizide. People with MODY may see intense blood sugar drops after taking as little as ¼ of the smallest dose of one of these sulfonylurea drugs. Some also respond very strongly to small doses of Prandin or Starlix.*

Treating MODY

Most forms of MODY are very much like Type 2 Diabetes in how they affect your body. Elevated blood sugars injure you slowly over many years, causing neuropathy, retinopathy, heart disease and the other ugly complications of diabetes.

The recommended treatment for MODY depends on the severity of the diabetes. Some people with MODY can maintain normal blood sugar levels by restricting carbohydrates. Others may be treated with very low doses of a sulfonylurea drug or tiny doses of insulin. Doctors assume you'd prefer a pill to shots, so they often suggest sulfonylurea drugs rather than insulin. But the insulin-stimulating drugs which are prescribed for people diagnosed with MODY may cause the relentless hunger and weight gain typical of these drugs and make them unpleasant to take.

Many people with MODY diabetes find that using very low doses of insulin at meal times gives them better control. Because they use very small doses, they rarely have to worry about dangerous hypos. Used in the tiny doses characteristic of MODY, insulin shouldn't cause weight gain.

If you suspect you have MODY and your doctor wants you to start insulin or a sulfonylurea drug, be sure to start at a very low dose. The starting dose of either a sulfonylurea drug or insulin appropriate for an insulin-resistant person with Type 2 Diabetes may be two to ten times higher than the dose that works well for a person with MODY. So the Type 2 starting dose may cause dramatic hypos in a person with MODY. When starting insulin, start with one unit and work up to the appropriate dose. Many people with MODY may do well with as little as 4-12 units a day. A typical Type 2 may use anywhere from 30 to 100 units.

There is anecdotal evidence that Byetta and Januvia may be very effective for people with some forms of MODY. If you are diagnosed

---

* To complicate this further, some people with MODY have very strong counterregulatory responses that push their blood sugar up as soon as it starts to go low. Instead of hypoing when they take a drug like Prandin, they may feel the jolt of counterregulatory hormones and see their blood sugar go up slightly. This can be difficult to interpret.

with MODY ask your doctor if you can try a course of Byetta.

If you suspect you have MODY diabetes and are of childbearing age, and if there is a strong history of diabetes in your spouse's family, consider genetic testing. A child who inherits two copies of the same MODY gene will be born with a severe form of diabetes, though given the rarity of MODY the chances of this occurring are extremely low. The chances are higher if you and your spouse share the same ethnic heritage.

Do It Yourself MODY Testing

If you suspect you have MODY but cannot get your insurer to pay for genetic testing there are two simple tests that may help you decide if it might be worth paying for testing.

The Renal Threshold Test for MODY-3

There is one useful home test you can do on your own that can help you determine if you may have MODY-3, the most common form of MODY. People with MODY-3 usually have an abnormally low renal threshold for glucose. This means they will spill glucose into urine at abnormally low blood sugar levels. Glucose usually appears in urine when blood sugar reaches 180 mg/dl. However, people with MODY-3 may find glucose in their urine when their blood sugar has only risen to 140 mg/dl.

You can test your own renal threshold by buying the urine test strips for glucose carried by most pharmacies. Test your urine one, two, and three hours after eating a meal that did not raise your one hour blood sugar over 150 mg/dl. If you have other symptoms characteristic of MODY and see glucose in your urine when your blood sugar did not go higher than 150 mg/dl, it is more likely that you do, in fact, have MODY-3.

People with MODY-3 are more likely to develop kidney disease, so if you find a low renal threshold, be sure your doctor monitors your kidney health. If there is a family history of kidney disease, be sure to have your kidneys evaluated by a nephrologist.

Sulfonylurea Sensitivity Test

You will need your doctor's help to perform this test. Explain that you believe you may have MODY and that people with MODY are extremely sensitive to sulfonylurea drugs. Then ask your doctor to prescribe for you the 1 mg dose of Amaryl. Amaryl is a sulfonylurea drug which is available as a generic and is part of the $4 generic prescription programs available at Wal-Mart and many other pharmacies.

Divide the 1 mg Amaryl pill into quarters using a sharp knife or a pill cutter. Be sure you have high carbohydrate foods on hand in case you have a strong response to the drug as a strong response can cause long lasting hypos. Take the one quarter tablet of Amaryl and eat a meal containing at least 30 grams of carbohydrates an hour later.

Test your blood sugar throughout the day. If your blood sugar stays flat or drops over the next eight hours, you are very sensitive to Amaryl and may indeed have MODY. If your blood sugar drops below 85 mg/dl eat high carbohydrate food every few hours. It may take up to eight hours until the drug stops affecting your blood sugars. You may find yourself ravenously hungry during the whole time it is active. Report your experience to your doctor. He will find it very unusual as people with Type 2 can usually take anywhere from 2 to 8 mg of Amaryl before seeing any significant blood sugar drop. This kind of sensitivity to a sulfonylurea drug is very suggestive that you have some form of MODY.

Insulin Sensitive Type 2 Diabetes

There is another possibility to consider if you have many of the symptoms described above but do not appear to have MODY.

There are other unidentified genetic defects besides the ones that are defined as MODY which cause *insulin sensitive* forms of Type 2 Diabetes. Though the genes at fault may be different than those causing MODY, the clinical manifestations may be the same: high blood sugars along with a lack of obesity, the development of gestational diabetes at a normal weight, and normal or high sensitivity to injected insulin.

All these suggest that your problem is a secretory defect rather than insulin resistance. For some reason, your beta cells are not secreting insulin when blood sugars start to rise. The treatment options for these kinds of Type 2 Diabetes are similar to the treatment options for MODY: Insulin after meals possibly combined with very low dose basal insulin, insulin stimulating drugs at low doses, or Byetta.

Whatever the cause for your diabetes the fundamental principle in treating it doesn't change. If you keep your blood sugar at normal levels, you should be able to avoid complications, and the best way to do that is to go easy on the carbohydrates and use only those drugs that have been proven to be safe.

Chapter Thirteen
Working with Doctors and Hospitals

Doctors who keep their knowledge about diabetes up-to-date can help you avoid a future filled with amputations, failing vision, and dialysis.

Not all doctors do. In fact, quite a few of the doctors you may encounter got their only formal training in diabetes care decades ago and the only "diabetes education" they've gotten since then has been provided by drug company representatives. Drug company "education" is nothing more than promotion for whatever is the newest, most expensive drug available for treating diabetes—education that does not mention dangerous side effects or that dismisses them as insignificant.

Other busy doctors get their only information about new diabetes treatments from skimming professional newsletters that report on the latest advances in patient care. These too tend to be heavily influenced by drug company press releases. They also adhere to the practice recommendations of the American Diabetes Association which downplay the dangers of high blood sugar and still favor the high carbohydrate/low fat diet which raises blood sugar and harms lipids.

Do You Have a Good Doctor?

Below you will find a list of questions you can use to evaluate the quality of the treatment you are getting from the medical professionals you are paying for your care. Use them to ensure that your doctor is a partner, not an obstacle, in your quest for normal health.

Does Your Doctor Support You in Your Efforts to Attain Normal Blood Sugars?

Be wary of any doctor who dismisses your concern about an abnormal blood sugar test because he thinks it isn't abnormal enough.

If your fasting blood sugar is over 105 mg/dl, or your post-meal blood sugars are routinely over 140 mg/dl two hours after eating, and your doctor tells you that this is normal or nothing to worry about, he is making it clear he is not aware of what mainstream medical practitioners now know about safe blood sugars. The same is true if your

A1c is over 6.5% and your doctor tells you that you don't need to worry about it. A doctor who considers elevated blood sugars "nothing to worry about" is likely to put roadblocks in the way of your getting better control or may lull you into a false sense of security.

You should not have to wait until you've lost all feeling in your toes, had your first retinal hemorrhage, or received your first lab test showing protein in your urine to have your doctor start taking your blood sugar seriously.

Does Your Doctor Order Appropriate Tests?

If you have not been diagnosed with diabetes but are at risk of developing it, the American Diabetes Association now recommends that your doctor should order a two hour Glucose Tolerance Test and diagnose you as diabetic if your blood sugar goes over 200 mg/dl at *any time*. Strong risk factors for diabetes would include being obese, having parents or siblings with diabetes, or having had gestational diabetes. If you have tested your blood sugar at home with a meter and seen several blood sugars over 140 mg/dl two hours after you have eaten, this is also a strong risk factor.

If your doctor believes you only need a fasting plasma glucose test or A1c test to rule out diabetes, he is out-of-date. As we saw earlier, fasting blood sugar often stays in the normal or mildly impaired range for years after post-meal blood sugars have risen into the diabetic range that causes complications.

The ADA warns doctors that the A1c test is not a valid test for diagnosing diabetes. This is because the A1c can return deceptively low values if a person is anemic or has certain genetic red blood cell variants.

Your doctor should also be sensitive to the issue of whether or not you have health insurance. If you don't, your doctor should be willing to suggest a less expensive test for diabetes than the expensive glucose tolerance test. For example, he may lend you a meter and suggest that you test your blood sugar one hour or two hours after eating a high carbohydrate meal and report the values to him.

If you live in a state where insurers are able to deny insurance to people diagnosed with diabetes, your doctor should be willing to help you figure out what is going on with your post-meal blood sugars and help you lower them, but avoid putting a formal diabetes diagnosis in your medical records. This is the *only* situation where relying on the fasting test for a diabetes diagnosis may benefit you.

Once you have been diagnosed with diabetes, your doctor should offer you an A1c test at least two times a year and discuss the test results with you. If your A1c is over 6.5% he should work with you to get your A1c under the American Association of Clinical Endocrinologists recommended 6.5% level, and if you prod him he should be willing to help you get it to under 6%. He should also test your urinary microalbumin, which is a measure of kidney health.

If you are on medications, your doctor should also order liver enzyme tests periodically to make sure that you aren't being injured by the drugs you are taking. If you are on Metformin, you should have your B-12 levels checked every few years.

Other signs your doctor is knowledgeable about diabetes are if he tests the pulses in your ankles to check the quality of your circulation and uses a filament or tuning fork to test the nerves in your feet. He should also refer you to an ophthalmologist for an eye exam each year. An ophthalmologist is a physician who specializes in the treatment of the eyes and is far more highly trained than the optometrists who do most eye exams.

If your doctor finds anything in your test results suggestive of early diabetic complications he should urge you to lower your blood sugars and work with you to find a safe drug regimen that will supplement the changes you make in your diet.

Does Your Doctor Prescribe Drugs Appropriately?

The practice recommendations published by the ultra-conservative American Diabetes Association state that Metformin should be the first drug that doctors prescribe to a patient with Type 2 Diabetes. That is because Metformin reduces insulin resistance and has a long safety record. Competent doctors should also know that the ER (extended release) form of Metformin does not cause as much stomach distress as the plain form. The cost of the ER version of the drug is the same as that of the regular so there is no reason not to prescribe the ER form.

Unfortunately, old fashioned doctors are also still prescribing sulfonylurea drugs as the first drug they give their diabetic patients, unaware that these drugs almost always cause hunger and weight gain that increases insulin resistance.

Other doctors give newly diagnosed patients whatever is the newest, most hyped, and most expensive drug often without understanding what it is that these new drugs do. Be cautious about a doctor who starts you on Byetta or Januvia before trying Metformin. These drugs do not lower insulin resistance and they often do not lower blood sugar. They are also extremely expensive.

Does Your Doctor Suggest Insulin When Oral Drugs Aren't Normalizing Blood Sugar?

If you have tried two or three oral medications and are still seeing high blood sugars, your doctor should suggest that you use insulin to get your blood sugars into the safe zone.

Insulin works, and modern insulins are much easier to use than those available in the past. If you have Type 2 Diabetes and your fasting blood sugar is still higher than 125 mg/dl with oral medications, your doctor should suggest Lantus or Levemir—assuming you have health insurance. If you don't have insurance, the cost of these insulins may be a problem. In that case, ask your doctor if you can use one of the cheaper regular human insulins. If using a basal insulin does not get you to your blood sugar goals, your doctor should be willing to refer you to an endocrinologist who can start you on meal-time insulin.

If You Are Not Getting Results or Are Having Troubling Side Effects Your Doctor Should Stop a Medication

One of the most worrisome things I observe in people posting on the Web is the number of people who are experiencing what are known to be dangerous side effects from commonly prescribed medications, whose doctors tell them to keep on taking them. Such side effects include muscle pain from statins, severe water retention with Avandia, and continual vomiting with Byetta. The first two symptoms can lead to permanent organ damage. The latter may point to pancreatitis.

Even worse, many patients report being put on expensive drugs that don't appear to do much for their blood sugars. If an expensive drug is not improving your blood sugar, there is no reason to take it. No drug will rejuvenate your beta cells if you are running blood sugars high enough to kill beta cells.

Does Your Doctor Know That Cutting Carbohydrates Is Safe and Effective?

Many people's doctors are still telling them to cut fat out of their diet, as if it were fat, rather than carbohydrates that raises blood sugar.

Some even warn patients that the low carbohydrate diet is dangerous, though even the American Diabetes Association revised its practice recommendations in 2008 to state that low carbohydrate diets are safe for people with diabetes.

Though he may not be enthusiastic about low carbohydrate dieting, your doctor should be aware that eliminating as much carbohydrate from your diet as possible and replacing that carbohydrate with fat is a safe and effective way to lower blood sugars. Your doctor should also know that the evidence now points to it being dietary carbohydrate that worsens lipids not fat, and that eating a low fat diet doesn't prevent heart disease.

Is Your Doctor's Staff Reasonable and Accessible?

Because family doctors are so overburdened, many of them have set up their practices so you don't deal with them directly but must talk to staff members when routine matters come up. These staff members may be highly trained nurse practitioners as competent as the doctor at handling routine requests or they may be LPN nurses with only a year of education beyond high school who nevertheless believe themselves competent to "screen" your call and who may decide not to pass your message on to the doctor.

It is very important to find a practice where the staff members you have to deal with are helpful, friendly, and, most importantly, able to pass your messages to your doctor without garbling them. If your doctor refers all his patients to a "diabetes nurse" for day-to-day case management, this is even more important. No matter how good your doctor is, you won't get good care if you have to go through a diabetes nurse who considers your call with a question about a high blood sugar frivolous or who believes that any A1c below 7.0% is "great control" no matter what kinds of numbers you are seeing after meals.

If your doctor expects a nurse to help you adjust your insulin doses, ask what that nurse's training has been. Ideally you'd like them to be a Certified Diabetes Educator. Find out, too, how long it has been since they've updated their training. There are a lot of "diabetes nurses" out there who are still treating patients with insulin regimens from twenty years ago—the kind that avoid hypos by allowing your blood sugar to rise dangerously high or which force you to eat a lot of carbohydrates to keep from going low.

What To Expect of a Good Doctor

Even with the very best doctor you are going to have to do a lot of the work of managing your diabetes yourself. Diabetes is the ultimate "do it yourself" condition. Keep up with the diabetes news yourself by tuning into Web discussion groups, blogs, or newsletters like Diabetes in Control. When you've done what you can on your own, ask your doctor to help you evaluate the information you have found. A good doctor should:

❖ Help you try out a new diabetes treatment you've heard about or explain to you why it isn't appropriate for you.

❖ Order appropriate tests after explaining to you what questions the tests can answer.

❖ Give you your actual test results, not a summary, and explain to you what these test results mean, answering any questions you may have about the test result.

❖ Give you a copy of your lab test results if you ask for them. You have a right to your test results and should always ask to have a copy made for you before you leave the office. Keep these test results in a file, as you may need to refer to them in the future if you change doctors. When doctors transfer records they often do not send all your old lab tests.

❖ Refer you to an appropriate specialist if something comes up that is not in their area of competence—and be honest about what that area of competence includes.

❖ Provide you with free samples of expensive new drugs he wants you to try if you do not have medical insurance, so you can find out if they work for you before you invest in them. If you don't have insurance or are in financial difficulty, your doctor or someone in his office should be able to explain to you how to sign up for drug company or state programs to help you get the drugs you need to preserve your health. He or his staff should also be willing to fill in any necessary paperwork you need for insurers or hardship drug support programs.

Diabetes at the Hospital or Nursing Home

If you have diabetes and are forced to go to a hospital, emergency room, or nursing home for any reason at all, you may find yourself plunged into a situation where well-intentioned but ignorant medical professionals do all they can to destroy your blood sugar control.

Because none of us know when we may be the victim of an accident or disease, every person with diabetes should prepare a "Medical Instruction Letter" signed by their primary care doctor or endocrinologist. This letter should describe in detail the diet and medications you should be given if you are hospitalized or put into a nursing home.

Hospitals and nursing homes still force patients with diabetes to eat the discredited low fat/high carbohydrate diet. They often use outdated insulin dosing schemes which guarantee that patients will experience very high post-meal blood sugars.

I have heard several stories about people put in nursing homes who had maintained excellent blood sugars before being institutionalized but were forced by the nursing home staff to eat very high carbohydrate meals and forbidden to set their own insulin doses even though they were mentally competent. The outdated care they received ruined their blood sugar control and in some cases contributed to their deaths.

Your Doctor No Longer Treats You at the Hospital

Over the past decade many hospitals have moved from the system where your own doctor visited you and dictated your treatment to a new system where a doctor called a "hospitalist" has complete control over your fate while you are hospitalized.

The hospitalist works only in the hospital and has no idea what treatment your regular doctor has prescribed for you. They may not even have access to your medical records. They specialize in critical care and are not likely to have been trained in the daily treatment of diabetes. If you are on insulin, they may forbid you to administer your own shots and put you at the mercy of nurses who use old-fashioned generic ways of dosing. You may be prohibited from testing your own blood sugar and discover that the meters the nurses are using are very old and very inaccurate.

Even worse, any doctor who sees the word "diabetes" on your chart may assume you have heart disease and order expensive tests completely unrelated to the reason that you went to the hospital because they assume that because you have diabetes any symptom you have—

including those resulting from accidents—must be a diabetic complication.

Don't Expect Anything You Say in the Hospital to Be Respected

Once you are signed into a hospital or nursing home, nothing you say will have any effect on your treatment, because the hospital and nursing home culture is one where only "Doctor's Orders" prevail.

If the hospitalist assigned your care believes that you should be eating a high carb/low fat diet, that's what you will be served. If they believe you should be given insulin on a sliding scale, that's what you'll be given. The only option you have in this situation is to sign out of the hospital with the words "against medical advice" put into your medical records. This is not feasible if you are in the hospital because of an accident or surgery.

Protect Yourself with a Doctor's Letter

Protect yourself with a letter which you draw up before you need it. You must have it put on your doctor's stationary and signed by your regular doctor. This letter should be entered into your medical records at your local hospital and ideally you should carry a copy or have your next of kin bring it to the hospital as soon as you are admitted.

Here's what you to do in your hospital letter:

❖ Have your doctor state that you are a highly compliant patient whose diabetes control is excellent and/or exemplary. State your A1c if it is under 6%.

❖ Have the doctor describe the diet that you should be placed on should you be hospitalized. If you are eating a low carbohydrate diet, it is not enough to say you are eating a "carbohydrate restricted" diet. My local hospital feeds people with diabetes what they describe as a "Carbohydrate Restricted Diabetes Diet." It provided 50 grams of carbohydrate per meal and no fat. The nutrition department refuses to serve any foods containing fat to a patient with a diabetes diagnosis. The amount of protein in the meals they provide for people with diabetes is very low, which would be a serious concern if you were there because you were undergoing surgery or healing from a wound.

❖ To avoid being put on this kind of dangerous "diabetes diet," you must have your doctor specify that you should be given a diet whose *percentage* of fat, protein, and carbohydrate per meal is specified.

❖ Have the doctor specify that if you are conscious you should be in charge of administering your own insulin and that you should be allowed to do your own blood sugar testing using your own equipment. Otherwise you may have your insulin and blood testing supplies removed at admission.

❖ If you are not conscious, you will be at the mercy of your local hospital staff. Discuss this problem with your doctor and ask for suggestions as to how it can be dealt with.

Appendix A
Convert Mg/dl to Mmol/L

Blood Sugar in mg/dl	Blood Sugar in mmol/L
20	1.1
50	2.8
60	3.3
70	3.9
85	4.7
90	5.0
100	5.5
108	6.0
110	6.1
120	6.7
125	7.0
140	7.7
150	8.3
180	18.0
200	11 .0
250	13.9
500	28.0

Table 5. Blood Sugar Equivalents: mg/dl to mmol/L

Appendix B
What Can You Eat When You are Cutting Carbohyrates?

Here are some foods that should be kind to your blood sugar, recommended by participants in various Web diet and diabetes support groups.

❖ **Pancakes**. Whey Protein powder can be cooked up to make pancakes. Add some strawberries or raspberries (frozen berries work very well) and some sugar free Maple Syrup and you've got a delicious breakfast. You'll find one recipe for a low carbohydrate protein pancake on Page 178.

❖ **Fauxtatoes**. A great substitute for mashed potatoes can be made by steaming or boiling cauliflower and pureeing it in a food processor with some cream or half and half, butter and salt. The result tastes much more like mashed potatoes than cauliflower.

❖ **Rolls**. Bake delicious rolls very similar to popovers using the "Magic Rolls" recipe from the Eades' *Low Carb Comfort Food Cookbook*. Make extra and freeze in a plastic bag. If you can't handle gluten, try making the "oopsies" egg and cream cheese rolls you'll find described on the **lowcarbfriends.com** discussion forum.

❖ **Veggies.** Here's a list of some healthy very low carbohydrate vegetables you should eat as much as possible. Romaine lettuce, Boston lettuce, red lettuce, mesclun mix, green beans, artichokes, avocado, asparagus, broccoli, Brussels sprouts, cabbage, cauliflower, collard greens, cucumbers, eggplant, kale, olives, spaghetti squash, spinach, Swiss chard, yellow summer squash, zucchini. The lower your carbohydrate intake, the better they will taste. Small amounts of fresh peppers and tomato work for most people, too, though they both contain some carbohydrate.

❖ **Soup.** Make homemade soups with broth and the vegetables listed above. Add a tablespoon of salsa to add flavor and variety. Cream and cheese soups are also delicious, especially if you add pureed cauliflower or broccoli instead of flour to thicken them.

❖ **Pasta.** Instead of using pasta with its over 50 grams of carbohydrate per tiny two ounce serving, pour your pasta sauces over lightly steamed zucchini strips you make with a vegetable peeler. Or use spaghetti squash. Shiritake noodles which contain a fiber called glucomannan are also very low in carbohydrate. Avoid pastas containing soy.

❖ **Sugar Substitute.** When baking, instead of Splenda powder, use DaVinci sugar free syrups for sweetening. Splenda powder contains maltodextrin, a sugar. In large portions, the carbohydrates in Splenda powder can add up. The DaVinci sugar free syrups contain no added sugars. These can be bought at Marshall's or TJ Maxx in the specialty food section. When baking, use a direct substitution: one teaspoon of sugar free syrup for one teaspoon of sugar. This works well for cheesecakes and custards.

❖ **Cookies.** You can make delicious very low carbohydrate macaroons with a recipe you'll find on Page 179. You can also make cookies using almonds ground very fine, but do not use almond flour if you are having trouble losing weight as it is very high in calories.

❖ **Snack Food.** Sunflower seeds in the shell make a good "finger food" snack. They are very low in carbohydrates and can take the place of chips while watching the game, etc. You can make snack chips by microwaving pepperoni slices or small pieces of American cheese on plastic wrap.

❖ **Candy.** Cream cheese fudge and coconut oil fudge make nice chocolate candy treats. You'll find recipes on Page 180.

❖ **Pizza.** When it's pizza time, get a meat/veggie combo and just eat the toppings. Some people make "meatza" using a thin lining of pepperoni as the bottom crust when they make pizza at home.

❖ **Chinese Restaurants.** Try Hot and Sour soup, teriyaki strips, crispy duck, ginger chicken or beef with string beans, and black bean sauce dishes. Ask for spareribs without any extra sauce. There are carbohydrates in all of these, so make this a rare treat.

❖ **Other Restaurants** Besides the obvious "chunk o' meat" entrees try the steak "bistro" salads or Caesar salads with grilled chicken or shrimp (not fried!). Avoid salads where you can't add the dressing yourself, as some chains will serve you bits of lettuce drenched in sugar as "salad." Stick with blue cheese, Parmesan peppercorn, ranch, oil and vinegar, or classic Italian dressing. Many flavored vinaigrettes are full of sugar. Many Steak House chains sprinkle MSG on their steaks which may improve flavor but leaves you ravenously hungry an hour later. Avoid those restaurants if you're trying to lose weight!

❖ **Nuts.** Almonds, walnuts, and pecans are low in carbohydrates and full of healthy oils. You can heat them on a cookie sheet for a few minutes with a coating of DaVinci flavored syrup to make them into a fancy treat.

❖ **Sinful Desserts.** Bake a low carbohydrate cheesecake. Use the Classic Philly 3 Step Cheesecake recipe. Substitute DaVinci sugar free syrup for the sugar and bake for a few minutes longer than usual. Instead of graham crackers, use a crushed nut crust made by chopping walnuts or almonds and pressing them into the pan.

❖ **Inventive Recipes.** Dana Carpender's book, *500 Low-Carb Recipes* is highly recommended.

Appendix C
Indispensable Low Carb Treats

Indispensable Almost No Carb Barbecue Sauce

This isn't a substitute for the "real thing," it's an improvement.

    3/8 cup vinegar

    1 1/2 cup tomato sauce. (One 15 oz can)

        (Don't use tomato sauce that has spices added to it)

    3 tablespoons Worcestershire Sauce

    1 1/2 tablespoon yellow hot dog mustard

    3/4 tablespoon Frank's Hot Sauce 3/4 tablespoon salt (optional)

    1 dash cayenne pepper

    3 teaspoons lemon juice

    1 1/2 teaspoon Liquid Smoke flavoring

    6 teaspoons Splenda

Add vinegar and all other ingredients except mustard to a sauce pan and heat to a medium temperature. Put mustard in a cup and slowly stir in a couple tablespoons of the mixture from the sauce pan until well blended. Stir the mustard mixture into the sauce in the pan.

Bring to a boil and lower heat. Let simmer for a few minutes. Let cool, then refrigerate.

Note: this sauce will taste a bit peculiar when it is still hot. Don't worry! Something magical happens when it sits in the fridge.

Serving: One half fluid ounce. Nutritional Info: <1 g carb, 0 g fat, 0 g protein, 6 calories.

Gravy

A product called "Not/Starch" from Expert Foods will thicken gravies, stews, and sauces without cornstarch or flour. It's all fiber. 1.7 g carb per teaspoon, 1.7 g fiber.

Another useful low carb thickener is Guar Gum which you can sometimes buy at health food stores or on the Web.

Jenny's Version of Garth's Macaroons

A modification of the recipe published by Garth Lamson. This is a truly low carb, low cal cookie that satisfies my need for a little after meal treat.

    1 1/3 cups unsweetened shredded coconut.

    1 tablespoon vanilla whey protein powder

    1/2 teaspoon salt

    1 tablespoon Splenda powder

    1 3/4 tablespoon DaVinci Amaretto sugar free syrup

        (You can use other flavors if you don't have this one)

    3/4 teaspoon Almond extract

    2 medium egg whites

Preheat oven to 325 degrees. Mix ingredients together in a bowl in order given. Drop by teaspoonfuls onto a lightly greased baking sheet. These do not spread out so you can put them close together.

Bake at 325 degrees for 20 minutes. Edges of cookies should be light brown. Remove from cookie sheet immediately.

Makes 24: Nutritional Info: ~1g carb, less than 1 g fiber, 1 g fat, 1 g protein, 17 calories.

Homemade Low Carb Pancakes

No hidden carbohydrates, great flavor, and a texture that is very close to the real thing. Add a teaspoon of cinnamon or pumpkin pie spice to the dry ingredients to make cinnamon spice pancakes.

    2.5 tablespoons or one scoop vanilla whey protein powder. Precision Engineered brand works better than some of the more expensive ones.

    3/4 teaspoon baking powder

    2 tablespoons water

    1 egg

    1 teaspoon vegetable oil (optional)

Mix dry ingredients in a bowl. Add the water, egg and oil in that order, stirring until each is incorporated and the batter is smooth. If batter is too thick to pour easily, add another tablespoon of water to thin it out. Fry in a pan or griddle with shortening as you would regular pancakes. Turn when bubbles appear at edges.

Serve with sugar free maple syrup.

Makes two pancakes. Nutritional Info: 1 g carb, 0 g fiber, 16 g protein, 14 g fat, 197 calories.

Almond or Hazelnut Cookies Made From Home Ground Nut Meal

Delicious, but relatively high in calories. So use this when you are in maintenance mode on your diet or if you need to boost your calories with nutritious foods.

    1 cup homemade hazelnut or almond flour
    1 tablespoon vanilla whey protein powder
    1/3 cup Splenda or 1/3 cup DaVinci sugar free syrup
        (Vanilla or amaretto flavors work well)
    1 egg white
    1/2 tablespoon almond extract

Preheat oven to 300 degrees. Line a cookie sheet with aluminum foil. To make nut flour, chop 1/3 of a pound of hazelnuts or almonds very fine. Stir in rest of ingredients in the order given. Using DaVinci syrup instead of powdered Splenda will cut the carbohydrate count of the total recipe by 11 grams but will make the cookies moister.

    Use a teaspoon to drop blobs 1/2 teaspoon in size on cookie sheet.
    Bake for 20 to 30 minutes until very lightly browned.
    Remove from oven and let cool. Then peel off foil.
    Makes 18. Nutritional Info: 1 g carb, 4 g fat, 1 g protein, 46 cal.

No Hidden Carb Fudge

This recipe makes 4 servings.

    2 ounces cream cheese (use the expensive kind with less starch filler)
    1 ounce baker's chocolate (the kind with no sugar.)
    1 tablespoon DaVinci Vanilla Sugar Free Syrup
        (or substitute 1 tablespoon Splenda and 1 teaspoon vanilla)
    2 tablespoon Cream

Melt the chocolate in the bottom of a greased small saucepan at low heat. Add the cream cheese and cream and stir in with the chocolate. Simmer. Add the DaVinci syrup (or Splenda and vanilla) and stir in. If it isn't sweet enough, add a tiny bit more syrup or Splenda until it tastes right. Cook until it starts to thicken. Take off the stove. Grease a small bowl or individual pie plate. Spoon fudge into bowl or plate. Chill in refrigerator until hard. Cut into 4 pieces. Enjoy!

    Makes 4 servings. Per serving: 2 g carb 1 g protein, 9.8 g fat, 99 calories.

Coconut Fudge

You can also make delicious "fudge" with this recipe.

2 tablespoons Virgin coconut oil

1 tablespoons cocoa powder (without milk or sugar)

1 teaspoon Splenda or DaVinci Sugar Free Syrup

Line a plate with plastic wrap. Melt the coconut oil in a cup in the microwave. Stir in cocoa powder and sweetener. Pour melted mixture onto plate, and refrigerate for fifteen minutes.

Makes 1 serving. Per serving: 3 g carb, 1 g protein, 14 g fat, 137 calories.

Low Carb Nut Muffin/Sweet Bread Mix

I discovered this recipe while trying to make a low carb pumpkin bread for Thanksgiving. To my surprise, the squash gave it a moist, non-rubbery, bread-like texture while contributing almost no pumpkin flavor. That makes the batter ideal for the muffins of your choice. The recipe below will make 9 muffins or 1 loaf of sweet bread.

7 1/2 ounces pumpkin or squash (one half of a 15 ounce can).

1 1/2 scoops (equivalent to 4 1/2 tablespoon) vanilla Protein Powder.

1 tablespoon vital wheat gluten.

1 tablespoon melted butter

1 egg

1 1/2 tablespoons DaVinci caramel (or vanilla) sugar free syrup

1/2 teaspoon baking powder

1/4 cup walnuts

1/4 cup grated coconut with no sugar added

Preheat Oven to 350 degrees. Grease bottom and sides of 9 muffin tin cups or a single bread pan. Mix all ingredients together in a big bowl in order given until completely blended. Pour batter into muffin cups or bread pan until it is about 1 inch deep.

Bake for 45 minutes or until a toothpick inserted into the muffin or bread comes up dry. Remove from pan and allow to cool. Cover with plastic wrap to retain moisture. Please note these are very moist and will develop mold after two days if you don't refrigerate them.

Makes 9 servings. Per 1 1/4 ounce serving: 3 g carb, 1 g fiber, 4g protein, 4 g fat, 64 calories.

Low Carb Yankee Chili

Here's another recipe the whole family will enjoy especially since these particular beans do not cause gas! One caution: *Do not eat soy if you have any thyroid issues. Soy worsens thyroid problems.*

10 ounces hamburger

1 can Eden brand Black Soy beans

(Buy them at health food stores. Don't use regular black beans.)

12 tablespoons strong chili powder. I use "Hard Times" brand Chili Mix.

14 ounces crushed peeled tomatoes (1/2 large can or 1 small can).

(Don't buy the seasoned varieties)

1 cup of water.

Fry up meat in skillet, when cooked, drain fat. Add tomatoes, beans, chili powder, and water. Simmer until thickened.

Makes 3 servings. Per serving: 22 g carb, 13 g fiber, 38 g protein, 20 g fat, 411 calories.

Very Low Carb Cocoa

This makes a nice substitute for coffee if you're trying to kick the habit, or just use it to keep warm in winter.

1 rounded teaspoon cocoa powder with no added milk or sugar.

1 teaspoon DaVinci Sugar Free Syrup of your choice.

(Kahuli Cafe is awesome. So is Amaretto.)

1 cup boiling water

Cream or half and half (as much as you'd put in coffee)

Boil the water. Put the cocoa powder into a cup and stir in the sugar free syrup until it makes a nice paste. Gradually stir in a tablespoon of boiling water. Then pour in the rest of the water. Fill almost to the top. Then lighten with the cream or half and half the way you would lighten coffee. You can use more cocoa to give it a stronger flavor.

One Serving. 2 g carb, 2 g fat, 27 calories when made with 1 tablespoon Half & Half. More calories with cream.

References

Chapter One: Normal Blood Sugar

The Genetic Basis of Type 2 Diabetes Mellitus: Impaired Insulin Secretion Versus Impaired Insulin Sensitivity. John E. Gerich. *Endocrine Reviews* 19 (4): 491-503

Is Reduced First-Phase Insulin Release the Earliest Detectable Abnormality in Individuals Destined to Develop Type 2 Diabetes? John E. Gerich. *Diabetes* 51:S117-S121, 2002

What is Normal Glucose? – Continuous Glucose Monitoring Data from Healthy Subjects. Professor J.S. Christiansen, presented at the Annual Meeting of the EASD.

Diagnosis and Classification of Diabetes Mellitus. American Diabetes Association. *Diabetes Care* 27:S5-S10, 2004

Chapter Two: How Diabetes Develops

You can read the history of how the American Diabetes Association set the arbitrary blood sugar levels used to diagnose diabetes at: **http://www.bloodsugar101.com/14046782.php**

The Natural History of Progression from Normal Glucose Tolerance to Type 2 Diabetes in the Baltimore Longitudinal Study of Aging. James B. Meigs et al. *Diabetes* 52:1475-1484, 2003

Mode of Onset of Type 2 Diabetes from Normal or Impaired Glucose Tolerance. Ele Ferrannini et al. *Diabetes* 53(1) 160-5 2003.

Prevalence of the Metabolic Syndrome Among US Adults: Findings from the Third National Health and Nutrition Examination Survey. Earl S. Ford et al. *JAMA*. 2002;287:356-359

Prevalence of Obesity, Diabetes, and Obesity-Related Health Risk Factors, 2001. Ali H. Mokdad et al. *JAMA* 2003;289:76-79

Down-Regulation of Diacylglycerol Kinase Delta Contributes to Hyperglycemia-Induced Insulin Resistance. Alexander V. Chibalin et al. *Cell* Vol 132, 375-386

Impaired Glucose Tolerance and Fasting Hyperglycaemia Have Different Characteristics. Davies MJ et al. *Diabet Med* 2000 Jun;17(6):433-40

Beta Cell Dysfunction and Glucose Intolerance: Results from the San Antonio Metabolism (SAM) Study. Gastaldelli A et al. *Diabetologia* 2004 Jan;47(1):31-9.

Gender Differences in the Prevalence of Impaired Fasting Glycaemia and Impaired Glucose Tolerance in Mauritius. Does Sex Matter? Williams JW et al. *Diabetic Medicine* 20 (11) 915 2003

Chapter Three: What Really Causes Diabetes?

ß-Cell Deficit and Increased ß-Cell Apoptosis in Humans with Type 2 Diabetes. Alexandra E. Butler et al. *Diabetes* 52:102-110, 2003 [The Mayo Patient Pancreas Autopsy Study]

Prevalence of Obesity, Diabetes, and Obesity-Related Health Risk Factors, 2001. Ali H. Mokdad et al. *JAMA* 2003;289:76-79

Do Common Plastics and Resins Carry Risks. Janet Raloff. *Science News*. Week of Sept. 29, 2007; Vol. 172, No. 13 (Rat photos.)

The Estrogenic Effect of Bisphenol-A Disrupts the Pancreatic β-Cell Function *In Vivo* and Induces Insulin Resistance. Alonso-Magdalena et al. *Environmental Health Perspectives* 113(January):106-112

Diabetes in Relation to Serum Levels of Polychlorinated Biphenyls and Chlorinated Pesticides in Adult Native Americans. Neculai Codru et al. *Environ Health Perspect.* 2007 October; 115(10): 1442-1447

Antidepressant Use Associated with Increased Type 2 Diabetes Risk. Caroline Cassels. Medscape.com. Report on research paper presented at 2007 ADA convention. **http://www.medscape.com/viewarticle/539078**

Glucose Tolerance in Adults after Prenatal Exposure to Famine. Ravelli AC, et al. *Lancet* 1998 Jan 17;351(9097):173-7

Insulin Resistance in the First-Degree Relatives of Persons with Type 2 Diabetes. Straczkowski M et al. *Med Sci Monit* 2003 May;9(5):CR186-90

Insulin Resistance in Children of Type 2 Parents who have Abnormal Mitochondria. Petersen KF et al. *New England J Med* 2004 Feb 12; 350(7);639-41

Molecular Mechanisms of Insulin Resistance in Humans and Their Potential Links With Mitochondrial Dysfunction. Katsutaro Morino et al. *Diabetes* 55:S9-S15, 2006

Chapter Four: Blood Sugar Level and Organ Damage

Increased Prevalence of Impaired Glucose Tolerance in Patients with Painful Sensory Neuropathy. Singleton, JR et al. *Diabetes Care* 24 (8) 1448-1453 2001

The Spectrum of Neuropathy in Diabetes and Impaired Glucose Tolerance. J. Sumner et al. *Neurology* 2003;60:108-111

Value of the Oral Glucose Tolerance Test in the Evaluation of Chronic Idiopathic Axonal Polyneuropathy. Charlene Hoffman-Snyder et al. *Arch Neurol.* 2006; 63:1075-1079

The Inflammatory Reflex. Kevin J. Tracey. *Nature* 420, 853-859 (19 December 2002)

Effect of an Intensive Glucose Management Protocol on the Mortality of Critically Ill Adult Patients. Krinsley, James. *Mayo Clinic Proc* Jan 2004, p. 992-1000

ß-Cell Death and Mass in Syngeneically Transplanted Islets Exposed to Short- and Long-Term Hyperglycemia. Montserrat Biarnés et al. *Diabetes* 51:66-72, 2002

Determinants of Glucose Toxicity and Its Reversibility in Pancreatic Islet Beta Cell Line, HIT-T15. Catherine E. Gleason et al. *Am J Physiol Endocrinol Metab* 279: E997-E1002, 2000

ADA Scientific Sessions: Retinopathy Found in Prediabetes. Elizabeth Thompson Beckley. *DOC News.* August 1, 2005. Volume 2 Number 8 p. 1

Prospective Study of Hyperglycemia and Cancer Risk. Pär Stattin et al. *Diabetes Care* 30:561-567, 2007

Fifty Percent of Patients with Coronary Artery Disease do Not Have Any of the Conventional Risk Factors. Futterman LG, Lemberg L.*Am J Crit Care.* 1998 May;7(3):240-4

Lipids, Risk Factors and Ischaemic Heart Disease. Castelli WP. *Atherosclerosis* 1996 Jul;124 Suppl:S1-9

Association of Hemoglobin A1c with Cardiovascular Disease and Mortality in Adults: The European Prospective Investigation into Cancer in Norfolk Kay-Tee Khaw et. al. *Annals of Internal Medicine* Vol 141, no 6, 413-420

Cardiac Steatosis in Diabetes Mellitus: A 1H-Magnetic Resonance Spectroscopy Study. McGavock JM et. al. *Circulation.* 2007 Sep 4;116(10):1170-5.

Postmeal Glucose Peaks at Home Associate with Carotid Intima-Media Thickness in Type 2 Diabetes. Katherine Esposito et. al. *J Clin Endo* doi:10.1210/jc.2007-2000

Glycemic Control and Coronary Heart Disease Risk in Persons With and Without Diabetes. The Atherosclerosis Risk in Communities Study. Elizabeth Selvin et. al. *Arch Intern Med.* 2005;165:1910-1916.

Post-Challenge Glucose Predicts Coronary Atherosclerotic Progression inn Non-Diabetic, Post-Menopausal Women P. B. Mellen et. al. *Diabetic Medicine* 24 (10), 1156-1159.

Chapter Five: Must You Deteriorate?

Controlling the Diabetes: Just What Can You Achieve? Roy Taylor, M.D.
http://www.medscape.com/viewarticle/460902_14

Diabetes Control and Complications Trial (DCCT)
http://diabetes.niddk.nih.gov/dm/pubs/control/

UK Prospective Diabetes Study (UKPDS)
http://www.dtu.ox.ac.uk/index.php?maindoc=/ukpds/

Long-Term Results of the Kumamoto Study on Optimal Diabetes Control in Type 2 Diabetic Patients. Motoaki Shichiri et al. *Diabetes Care* Vol 23 Sup 2, 2000

Effects of Duration of Type 2 Diabetes Mellitus on Insulin Secretion. Farhad Zangeneh, Puneet S. Arora et al. *Endocr Pract.* 2006;12:388-393

Chapter Six: How to Lower Blood Sugar

Dr. Bernstein's Diabetes Solution: The Complete Guide to Achieving Normal Blood Sugars, Third Ed., Richard K. Bernstein. Little Brown, New York, 2007, ISBN 978-0316167161. P. 259 [No need for alcohol swabbing]

Protein Power. Michael R. Eades and Mary Dan Eades, Bantam Books, 1997. ISBN: 978-0553574753

The earliest references to The 5% Club is found in this alt.support.diabetes posting: http://groups.google.com/group/alt.support.diabetes/browse_frm/thread/40c55ce608d68b4e/

AACE "Medical Guidelines for Clinical Practice for the Management of Diabetes Mellitus.2007" http://www.aace.com/pub/guidelines/

Evolution in the American Diabetes Association Standards of Care. John B. Buse, *Clinical Diabetes* 21:24-26, 2003

Chapter Seven: Making the Diet Work

Comparison of the Atkins, Ornish, Weight Watchers, and Zone Diets for Weight Loss and Heart Disease Risk Reduction. A Randomized Trial. Michael L. Dansinger et al. *JAMA.* 2005;293:43-53

Comparison of the Atkins, Zone, Ornish, and LEARN Diets for Change in Weight and Related Risk Factors Among Overweight Premenopausal Women. Christopher D. Gardner et al. *JAMA.* 2007;297:969-977

A Low-Carbohydrate, Ketogenic Diet to Treat Type 2 Diabetes. William S Yancy, Jr. et al. *Nutr Metab* (Lond). 2005; 2: 34.

Effect of a High-Protein, Low-Carbohydrate Diet on Blood Glucose Control in People with Type 2 Diabetes. Mary C. Gannon et al. *Diabetes* 53:2375-2382, 2004

Effect of a Low-Carbohydrate Diet on Appetite, Blood Glucose Levels, and Insulin Resistance in Obese Patients with Type 2 Diabetes. Guenther Boden et al. *Ann Intern Med* 2005 Mar 15;142(6):403-11

The Effects of Low-Carbohydrate Versus Conventional Weight Loss Diets in Severely Obese Adults: One-Year Follow-up of a Randomized Trial. Stern L et al. *Ann Intern Med.* 2004 May 18; 140(10):778-85

Lasting Improvement of Hyperglycaemia and Bodyweight: Low-Carbohydrate Diet in Type 2 Diabetes. A Brief Report. Nielsen JV et al. *Ups J Med Sci.* 2005;110(2):179-83

Good Calories, Bad Calories. Gary Taubes. Knopf. New York, 2007. ISBN: 978-1400040780

Chapter Eight: Diabetes Drugs

The FDA mandated "**Prescribing Information**" for all drugs can be found in the *Physicians Desk Reference* (PDR) or search for it on the Web. Your pharmacist can also give you a copy.

Diabetes Prevention Program Research Group; Reduction in the Incidence of Type 2 Diabetes with Lifestyle Intervention or Metformin. *N E J of Med*, Vol 346:393-403 Feb 7, 2002 Number 6

Mechanism of Metformin Action in Obese and Lean Noninsulin-Dependent Diabetic Subjects. DeFronzo RA, et al. *J Clin Endocrinol Metab* 1991 Dec;73(6):1294-301

Metformin Increases AMP-Activated Protein Kinase Activity in Skeletal Muscle of Subjects with Type 2 Diabetes. Nicolas Musi et al. *Diabetes* 51: 2074-2081

Effect of Pioglitazone Compared with Metformin on Glycemic Control and Indicators of Insulin Sensitivity in Recently Diagnosed Patients with Type 2 Diabetes. Imre Pavo et al. *J Clin Endo & Metab* Vol. 88, No. 4 1637-1645

Incidence of Lactic Acidosis in Metformin Users. Stang M et al. *Diabetes Care.* Jun 1999, 22(6) p925-7

Risk of Fatal and Nonfatal Lactic Acidosis with Metformin Use in Type 2 Diabetes Mellitus: Systematic Review and Meta-Analysis. Salpeter SR et al. *Arch Intern Med* 2003 Nov 24;163(21):2594-602.

Effects of Short-Term Treatment with Metformin on Serum Concentrations of Homocysteine, Folate and Vitamin B12 in Type 2 Diabetes Mellitus: A Randomized, Placebo-Controlled Trial. Wulffele MG et al. *J Intern Med* 2003 Nov;254(5):455-63.

Effects of the Alpha-Glucosidase Inhibitor Acarbose on the Development of Long-Term Complications in Diabetic Animals: Pathophysioloical and Therapeutic Implications. Creutzfeldt W. *Diabetes Metab Res* rev. 1999 15(4):289-96

STOP-NIDDM Trial Research Group. Acarbose for Prevention of Type 2 Diabetes Mellitus: the STOP-NIDDM Randomised Trial. Chiasson JL et al. *Lancet* 2002 Jun 15;359 (9323):2072-7

Dose-Response Relation Between Sulfonylurea Drugs and Mortality in Type 2 Diabetes Mellitus: A Population-Based Cohort Study. Scot H. Simpson, et al. *CMAJ* January 17, 2006; 174

Preventing Diabetes - No DREAM Solution. http://www.diabetesincontrol.com/results.php?storyarticle=4766

Scientist Says Executive of Avandia Firm Tried to Bully. Study by Researcher Tied Drug to Heart Ills. Diedtra Henderson, *Boston Globe*. June 7, 2007

F.D.A. Review Criticizes Diabetes Drug and Maker, Gardiner Harris. *New York Times.* July 26, 2007

Thiazolidinediones and Heart Failure: A Teleo-Analysis. Sonal Singh et al. *Diabetes Care,* published online ahead of print May 29, 2007

Effects of Pioglitazone Versus Diet and Exercise on Metabolic Health and Fat Distribution in Upper Body Obesity. Samyah Shadid, MD and Michael D. Jensen, MD. *Diabetes Care* 26:3148-3152, 2003

Thiazolidinedione-Associated Congestive Heart Failure and Pulmonary Edema. Kermani A, Garg A. *Mayo Clin Proc* 2003 Sep;78(9):1088-91

Considerations for Management of Fluid Dynamic Issues Associated with Thiazolidinediones. Hollenberg NK. *Am J Med.* 2003 Dec 8;115 Suppl 8A:111S-115S

Glitazone Use May Be Associated with Macular Edema in Diabetics. Karla Harby. http://www.medscape.com/viewarticle/464732

Rosiglitazone-Induced Granulomatous Hepatitis. Dhawan M, Agrawal R et al. *J Clin Gastroenterol* May-Jun 2002, 34(5) p582-4

Hepatotoxicity of the Thiazolidinediones. Tolman KG, Chandramouli. *J. Clin Liver Dis* May 2003, 7(2) p369-79

Type 2 Diabetes, Thiazolidinediones: Bad to the Bone? Watts NB et al. *J Clin Endocrinol Metab* 2006;91:3276-3278

Diabetes, TZDs, and Bone: A Review of the Clinical Evidence. Ann V. Schwartz. *PPAR Res.* 2006; 2006: 24502

Avandia Researchers Find Reason Behind Bone Fracture, Osteoporosis Side Effects. Dec. 3, 2007. http://www.newsinferno.com/archives/2123

BYETTA® Study Showed Sustained Blood Glucose Control Over Three Years in People with Type 2 Diabetes. Lilly Amylin PR Newswire press release. June 25, 2007

FDA Warning on Byetta and Pancreatitis: http://www.fda.gov/medwatch/safety/2007/safety07.htm#Byetta

Anecdotal experience with Byetta Side effects http://www.diabetesmonitor.com/byettafaq.htm

Circulating CD26 [DPP-4] Is Negatively Associated with Inflammation in Human and Experimental Arthritis. Nathalie Busso et al. *Am J Pathol* 2005;166:433-442

Studies of DPP-4 gene function: http://www.ihop-net.org/UniPub/iHOP/bng/87784,html

A Role for Dipeptidyl Peptidase IV in Suppressing the Malignant Phenotype of Melanocytic Cells, Umadevi V. Wesleya et al. *J. Exp. Med* Volume 190, Number 3, August 2, 1999 311-322

Dipeptidyl Peptidase IV (DPPIV) Inhibits Cellular Invasion of Melanoma Cells. Pethiyagoda CL et al. *Clin Exp Metastasis* 2001, 18:391-400

Prolonged Survival and Decreased Invasive Activity Attributable to Dipeptidyl Peptidase IV Overexpression in Ovarian Carcinoma. Hiroaki Kajiyama et al. *Cancer Research* 62, 2753-2757, May 15, 2002

Chapter Nine: Insulin

Think Like a Pancreas: A Practical Guide to Managing Diabetes with Insulin. Gary Scheiner. Marlowe, 2004. ISBN: 1569244367

Dr. Bernstein's Diabetes Solution, op. cit.

Using Insulin, Everything You Need for Success With Insulin. John Walsh et al. Torrey Pines Press ISBN: 978-1884804854

Chapter Ten: Supplements and Healing Foods

A Hydroxychalcone Derived from Cinnamon Functions as a Mimetic for Insulin in 3T3-L1 Adipocytes. Jarvill-Taylor KJ et al. DJ. *J Am Coll Nutr* 20: 327-336, 2001

Cinnamon Extract (Traditional Herb) Potentiates in Vivo Insulin-Regulated Glucose Utilization Via Enhancing Insulin Signaling in Rats. Qin B et al. *Diabetes Res Clin Pract* 2003 Dec;62(3):139-48

Elevated Intakes of Supplemental Chromium Improve Glucose and Insulin Variables in Individuals with Type 2 Diabetes. RA Anderson et al. *Diabetes*, Vol 46, Issue 11 1786-1791

Insulin Potentiating Factor and Chromium Content of Selected Foods and Spices. Khan A, Bryden et al. *Biol Trace Elem Res.* 1990 Mar;24(3):183-8

Chromium, Glucose Intolerance and Diabetes. Richard A. Anderson, *Journal of the American College of Nutrition*, Vol. 17, No. 6, 548-555 (1998)

Role of Chromium Supplementation in Indians with Type 2 Diabetes Mellitus. Ghosh D et al. *J Nutr Biochem* 2002 Nov;13(11):690-697

Glucose and Insulin Responses to Dietary Chromium Supplements: A Meta-Analysis. Althuis et al. *Am J Clin Nutr* 2002 Jul;76(1):148-55

Chromium (III) Tris (Picolinate) is Mutagenic at the Hypoxanthine (Guanine) Phosphoribosyltransferase Locus in Chinese Hamster Ovary Cells. Stearns DM et al. *Mutat Res* (Netherlands), Jan 15 2002, 513(1-2) p135-42

Nutritional Supplement Chromium Picolinate Causes Sterility and Lethal Mutations in Drosophila Melanogaster. Hepburn DD et al. *Proc Natl Acad Sci* Apr 1 2003, 100(7) p3766-71.

Chromium Picolinate for Reducing Body Weight: Meta-Analysis of Randomized Trials.M H Pittler et al. *International Journal of Obesity* April 2003, Volume 27, Number 4, Pages 522-529

MRC/BHF Heart Protection Study of Antioxidant Vitamin Supplementation in 20,536 High-Risk Individuals: A Randomised Placebo-Controlled Trial. Heart Protection Study Collaborative Group. *Lancet* Jul 6 2002, 360(9326) p23-33

Vitamin C and Hyperglycemia in the European Prospective Investigation into Cancer—Norfolk (EPIC-Norfolk) study: a Population-based Study. Sargeant LA et al. *Diabetes Care* (United States), Jun 2000, 23(6) p726-32

Occupational Social Class, Educational Level and Area Deprivation Independently Predict Plasma Ascorbic Acid Concentration: A Cross-Sectional Population Based Study in the Norfolk Cohort of the European Prospective Investigation Into Cancer (EPIC-Norfolk). Shohaimi S et al. *Eur J Clin Nutr* Mar 31 2004

Double-Blind, Randomised Study of the Effect of Combined Treatment With Vitamin C And E on Albuminuria in Type 2 Diabetic Patients. Gaede P, Poulsen et al. *Diabet Med* Sep 2001, 18(9) p756-60

Mortality in Randomized Trials Of Antioxidant Supplements for Primary and Secondary Prevention: Systematic Review and Meta-Analysis. Bjelakovic G, Nikolova D et al. *JAMA* 2007 Feb 28;297(8):842-57

A Miricle Diabetes Cure. Gretchen Becker.
http://www.healthcentral.com/diabetes/c/5068/19892/miracle-cure/

Dr. Bernstein's Diabetes Solution, op. cit. p. 246. Vanadyl Sulfate.

Oral Administration of RAC-Alpha-Lipoic Acid Modulates Insulin Sensitivity in Patients with Type-2 Diabetes Mellitus: A Placebo-Controlled Pilot Trial. Jacob S, Ruus P et al. *Free Radic Biol Med* (United States), Aug 1999, 27(3-4) p309-14

Oral Treatment With Alpha-Lipoic Acid Improves Symptomatic Diabetic Polyneuropathy. The SYDNEY Trial. Dan Ziegler et al. *Diabetes Care* 29:2365-2370, 2006

Alpha-Lipoic Acid: A Multifunctional Antioxidant that Improves Insulin Sensitivity in Patients with Type 2 Diabetes. Evans JL, Goldfine ID. *Diabetes Technol Ther* Autumn 2000, 2(3) p401-13

Magnesium Intake and Risk of Type 2 Diabetes in Men And Women. Ruy Lopez-Ridaura et al. *Diabetes Care* 27:134-140, 2003

Dietary Magnesium Intake in Relation to Plasma Insulin Levels and Risk of Type 2 Diabetes in Women. Lopez-Ridaura R et al. *Diabetes Care* 27:59-65, 2003

Fructose, Weight Gain, and the Insulin Resistance Syndrome. Sharon S. Elliott et al. *American Journal of Clinical Nutrition* Vol 76 No. 5 911-922, 2002

Experimental Studies on the Role of Fructose in the Development of Diabetic Complications. Sakai M, Oimomi M et al. *J Med Sci* (Japan), Dec 2002, 48(5-6) p125-36

The Whole Soy Story: The Dark Side of America's Favorite Health Food. Kaayla T. Daniel, Ph.D. NewTrends Publishing, Inc, 2005. ISBN-13: 978-0967089751

Use uf Soy Protein Supplement and Resultant Need for Increased Dose of Levothyroxine. Bell DS et al. *Endocr Pract* 2001 May-Jun;7(3):193-4

The Role of Vitamin D and Calcium in Type 2 Diabetes. A Systematic Review and Meta-Analysis. Anastassios G. Pittas et al. *J Clin Endo & Metab* Vol. 92, No. 6 2017-2029

Benfotiamine Prevents Macro- and Microvascular Endothelial Dysfunction and Oxidative Stress Following a Meal Rich in Advanced Glycation End Products in Individuals With Type 2 Diabetes. Alin Stirban, et al. *Diabetes Care* 29:2064-2071, 2006

Benfotiamine Blocks Three Major Pathways of Hyperglycemic Damage and Prevents Experimental Diabetic Retinopathy. Hans-Peter Hammes et al. *Nature Medicine* 9, 294-299 (2003)

Benfotiamine in the Treatment of Diabetic Polyneuropathy—A Three-Week Randomized, Controlled Pilot Study (BEDIP Study). Haupt E, Ledermann et al. *Int J Clin Pharmacol Ther* 2005 Feb;43(2):71-7

Oral Administration of RAC-Alpha-Lipoic Acid Modulates Insulin Sensitivity in Patients with Type-2 Diabetes Mellitus: A Placebo-Controlled Pilot Trial. Jacob S et al. *Free Radic Biol Med* Aug 1999, 27(3-4) p309-14

Alpha-Lipoic Acid: A Multifunctional Antioxidant that Improves Insulin Sensitivity in Patients with Type 2 Diabetes. Evans JL, Goldfine. *Diabetes Technol Ther* Autumn 2000, 2(3) p401-13

Chapter Eleven: Exercise

Effects of Exercise on Glycemic Control and Body Mass in Type 2 Diabetes Mellitus: A Meta-analysis of Controlled Clinical Trials. Normand G. Boulé, et al. *JAMA.* 2001;286:1218-1227.

Intensity and Amount of Physical Activity in Relation to Insulin Sensitivity: The Insulin Resistance Atherosclerosis Study. Elizabeth J. Mayer-Davis et al. *JAMA.* 1998;279:669-674.

Target Heart Rate. American Heart Association.
http://www.americanheart.org/presenter.jhtml?identifier=4736

Some Long-Term Sequelae of Poorly Controlled Diabetes that are Frequently Undiagnosed, Misdiagnosed or Mistreated. Richard K. Bernstein
http://www.diabetes-book.com/articles/poorly_controlled_diabetes.shtml

Carpal Tunnel May Predict Diabetes (WebMD)
http://diabetes.webmd.com/news/20060822/carpal-tunnel-predict-diabetes

Thickness of the Supraspinatus and Biceps Tendons in Diabetic Patients. Mujde Akturk et al. *Diabetes Care* 25:408, 2002

Dr. Bernstein's Diabetes Solution, op. cit. 214-222.

Using Pedometers to Increase Physical Activity and Improve Health: A Systematic Review. Dena M. Bravata, MD et. al. *JAMA* 2007;298(19):2296-2304

Keeping it Off: Winning at Weight Loss. Robert H. Olson and Susan C. Colvin. Gilliland, 1989. ISBN: 0671532944

Chapter Twelve: Is it Really Type 2

Latent Autoimmune Diabetes Of Adulthood: Unique Features that Distinguish It From Types 1 and 2. Fadi Nabhan et al. *Postgraduate Medicine* Vol 117, No 3, Mar 2005

Identification of MODY: The Implications for Holly. Jo Dalton, Maggie Shepherd. *Journal of Diabetes Nursing* Jan, 2004

Determinants of the Development of Diabetes (Maturity-Onset Diabetes of the Young- in Carriers of HNF-1{alpha} Mutations. Evidence for Parent-of-Origin Effect. Tomasz Klupa, et al. *Diabetes Care* 25:2292-2301, 2002

Altered Insulin Secretory Responses to Glucose In Diabetic and Nondiabetic Subjects with Mutations in the Diabetes Susceptibility Gene MODY3 on Chromosome 12MM. Byrne et al. *Diabetes* Vol 45, Issue 11 1503-1510

Assessment of Insulin Sensitivity in Glucokinase-Deficient Subjects. Clement K et al. *Diabetes Care* 25:2292-2301, 2002

Genes and Diabetes: Molecular and Clinical Characterization of Mutations in Transcription Factors. Timothy M. Frayling et al. *Diabetes* Vol. 50, Sup 1, Feb 2001

Genetic Types of Diabetes Including MODY (UK - Exeter Research & Testing) http://www.projects.ex.ac.uk/diabetesgenes/

Diagnosis and Management of Maturity-Onset Diabetes of the Young. Timsit, Jose et al. *Treat in Endo* 4(1):9-18, 2005 (Contains finding that parents carrying gene may not have been diagnosed)

Chapter Thirteen: Workng with Doctors and Hospitals

American Association of Clinical Endocrinologists: Most Recent AACE Guidelines. http://www.aace.com/pub/guidelines/

Dr. Bernstein's Diabetes Solution. op cit. Appendix B p. 462. Sample doctor letter.

Medical research is surprisingly silent on the topic of the competence of medical practitioners. This chapter draws mostly on thousands of anecdotal reports posted by people with diabetes who have achieved excellent control.

Appendix B: What Can You Eat?

The Low-Carb Comfort Food Cookbook. Michael R. Eades et al.Wiley, 2002. ISBN: 978-0471267577. Magic Rolls are on P. 22.

500 Low-Carb Recipes: 500 Recipes from Snacks to Dessert, That the Whole Family Will Love. Dana Carpender. Fair Winds Press, 2002. ISBN: 978-1931412063

Google Advanced Group Search: http://groups.google.com/advanced_search

Appendix C: Indispensable Low Carb Treats

Garth Lamson's low carb recipes can be found at:
http://lamsonadventures.com/recipes/atkins.html

Acknowledgements

This book grew out of years of daily interaction with hundreds of people active in the online diabetes community, each one of whom has contributed something valuable. My thanks to all!

I have learned a great deal from the many people who have posted informative messages on the alt.support.diabetes newsgroup over the years. Special thanks to those who post under the names, Alan S., Alice Faber, Annette, Chakolate, Chris Malcolm, GysdeJongh, Jefferson a.k.a. Frank Roy, Julie Bove, Loretta, Mack, Nicky, Old Al, OtterCritter, Ozgirl, Priscilla H Ballou, Quentin Grady, Ratty, Susan, W. Baker, Ted Rosenberg, and Wes Groleau.

Steve Freed does a great job keeping the diabetes community informed of the latest medical news with his Diabetesincontrol.com newsletter. I'm also grateful to him for making possible Dr. Bernstein's free teleconferences.

Thanks to Manny Hernandez for creating Tudiabetes.com, a nurturing online community for people with diabetes. Thanks to David and Elizabeth Edelman whose Diabetesdaily.com headline service provides quick access to a long list of diabetes blogs.

I am fortunate to have Gretchen Becker as a friend. She keeps me grounded when I indulge in too much speculation and comes up with helpful citations I've missed.

My gratitude to Dr. Richard K. Bernstein is in a class by itself. I picked up his book, *Dr. Bernstein's Diabetes Solution*, the day I was diagnosed in 1998. What I read there contradicted everything my doctors told me. But unlike what they told me, his advice worked. It was radical back then, by now it is almost mainstream. His legacy will be a generation of people with diabetes who do not develop the diabetic complications caused by tragically flawed medical advice.

Words are not enough to thank my life partner, Peter Atwood, for all that he does, including — let's be honest here — bringing home far too much excellent pastry.

Index